THE
PEOPLE'S
HOSPITAL
BOOK

By Ronald Gots, M.D., Ph.D.

THE TRUTH ABOUT MEDICAL MALPRACTICE
CARING FOR YOUR UNBORN CHILD

THE PEOPLE'S HOSPITAL BOOK

How to
· Increase your comfort and safety
· Deal with nurses and doctors
· Obtain the best total care.

RONALD GOTS, M.D., Ph.D.
and
ARTHUR KAUFMAN, M.D.

Foreword by Jonathan E. Fielding, M.D., M.P.H.
Massachusetts Commissioner of Public Health

CROWN PUBLISHERS, INC., NEW YORK

ACKNOWLEDGMENTS

Our deepest appreciation to Marian Behrman, our editor, whose infectious enthusiasm and ongoing dialogue was a constant source of inspiration. She made this book possible. Our thanks to Rosemary Baer, our copy editor. Her precision and literary ability added clarity and crispness for our readers. Finally, our sincere thanks to Bonnie Waldman, Diana L. Dean, Dee Edwards, and Gail Green Grob, CSW, ACSW, for their excellent technical assistance.

Inquiries should be addressed to Crown Publishers, Inc., One Park Avenue,
New York, N.Y. 10016
Printed in the United States of America. Published simultaneously in Canada by
General Publishing Company Limited

Book Design: Huguette Franco

Library of Congress Cataloging in Publication Data

Gots, Ronald E
The people's hospital book.

1. Hospitals.   2. Hospital care.   3. Hospital
patients.   I. Kaufman, Arthur, joint author.
II. Title.
RA963.G67   362.1′1   78-17994
ISBN 0-517-53323-5

FOREWORD

Most people, including health care professionals, have two reactions to hospitals—on the one hand they are comforted by their imposing physical presence, their proximity and reputation; yet on the other, most people are scared at the prospect of themselves or someone in their family entering a hospital as a patient. Hospitals are big business; they are hierarchical institutions staffed by a diversified group of specialized personnel and with a large number of written and unwritten rules. Because so many people are routinely involved in the care of those who are hospitalized, patients infrequently feel they are receiving personalized attention. Patients may even be unsure who is the physician with primary responsibility for their care. Thus, a hospital stay can become an unnecessarily negative or demoralizing experience unless the potential patient is prepared.

Despite the importance to the individual of decisions made surrounding hospitalization, many Americans lack sufficient familiarity with the system to make well-informed choices. In addition to fear, the need for hospital care generates anxiety, frustration, concern for dependents, and worry about possible economic consequences. In these tension-filled situations often the crucial decisions—the choice of a hospital, selection of a surgeon, assessment of necessary consultants—are not made by patients or their families. Drs. Gots and Kaufman have set themselves the difficult task of dissecting the hospital experience in striving to make their readers informed patients. They have done their careful homework by visiting a large cross section of America's hospitals and querying many patients. The authors' empathetic but in depth description of how a hospital operates can help any prospective patient (and who isn't one?) make better decisions about where, how, and from whom to get the most out of the medical care system. At the very least, the careful reader will be more willing and able to assume responsibility for important decisions that they should be making and not leaving to chance.

Jonathan E. Fielding, M.D., M.P.H.
Massachusetts Commissioner of Public Health

Contents

Foreword   v

Introduction   1

Chapter **1**   WHY CHOOSING A HOSPITAL IS ONE OF THE
                  MOST IMPORTANT DECISIONS YOU MAY EVER
                  MAKE   4
                  • You may have more choices than you think
                  • What will determine your decision

Chapter **2**   ASSESSING YOUR NEEDS   15
                  • How to assess your needs
                  • How to protect yourself from the most
                    dangerous aspect of surgery—anesthesia
                  • How to judge the competence of your surgeon
                  • Which hospital for your child—a particularly
                    critical decision

Chapter **3**   WHICH HOSPITAL IS BEST FOR YOUR NEEDS   36

- Large versus small hospitals
- University hospitals
- Other teaching hospitals
- Nonteaching hospitals
- How to find the "best" hospital
- When to check out your local hospital situation

Chapter **4**   THE EMERGENCY DEPARTMENT: HOW TO CUT
DOWN·ON YOUR FRUSTRATIONS   44

- Planning ahead for emergencies
- How to decide whom to call
- Understanding the inner workings of the
  emergency department
- How to assess the kind of attention you
  deserve
- What to do if you are dissatisfied with
  treatment
- What the relative or friend can do

Chapter **5**   HOSPITALS AWAY FROM HOME   63

- Finding the best hospitals
- Arranging a transfer
- Preplanning for travel away from home

Chapter **6**   EXPEDITING YOUR ADMISSION TO THE
HOSPITAL   70

- Things to do before you go
- What to take
- Speeding the admission process
- The emergency admission

Chapter **7**   UNDERSTANDING THE NURSING STAFF AND
HOW IT CAN BENEFIT YOU   78

- A who's who of nursing

Chapter **8**   YOU AND THE NURSES: ACHIEVING A MORE
EFFECTIVE RELATIONSHIP   84

- How to increase your comfort and safety
- How to assess your needs realistically

- Minor and major complaints and how to
  handle them
- Special care nurses
- When to use and when not to use private-duty
  nurses

Chapter **9** THE PHYSICIAN STAFF AND HOW IT AFFECTS
YOU PERSONALLY   96

- Why the chain of command is important to
  you
- How to make sure a complaint or a question
  will count
- The role of consultants
- The setup of the teaching hospital

Chapter **10** PHYSICIAN CARE IN THE HOSPITAL: THE
BENEFITS OF BEING AWARE AND INVOLVED   109

- Who is your doctor? Do you really know?
- How to assure that your health care is well
  coordinated
- How and when to change doctors

Chapter **11** UNDERSTANDING PROCEDURES AND
EQUIPMENT: A GOOD WAY TO LESSEN YOUR
ANXIETY   122

- Laboratory studies and procedures
- Modern techniques and equipment

Chapter **12** LABOR AND DELIVERY: WHY ALTERNATE
METHODS OF CHILDBIRTH NECESSITATE A
MORE KNOWLEDGEABLE CONSUMER   131

- Home versus hospital—the determining criteria
- How to get the best of both worlds
- New alternatives hospitals are offering
- Finding a physician who shares your goals
- Drugs—how to avoid the quiet trap
- What to expect in labor and delivery
- Cesarean section—when is it necessary?

Chapter **13** SURGERY: GETTING THROUGH IT WITH THE LEAST STRESS AND SPEEDING YOUR RECOVERY 143

- Preplanning
- Second opinions
- What to expect before and after the operation
- Self-help for postsurgical discomfort
- Private-duty nursing and the postsurgical patient
- Assisting with your recovery

Chapter **14** SPECIAL CARE UNITS: WHAT THEY CAN DO FOR YOU AND WHAT YOU CAN DO FOR A LOVED ONE 163

- Shock-trauma or critical care centers
- Burn centers
- Neurological injury centers
- Intensive care units
- Coronary care units
- Renal dialysis centers
- Neonatal intensive care units
- The family's role in helping patients in special care units

Chapter **15** SOME PRACTICAL ANSWERS TO QUESTIONS ABOUT DAILY HOSPITAL LIFE 171

- Visitors and visiting hours
- Semiprivate versus private—how do you choose?
- Patient orientation
- Hospital food
- Special patient education
- Books and arts-and-crafts services
- Relatives sleeping in
- Gifts

Chapter **16** PREPARING YOUR CHILD FOR THE HOSPITAL 180

- Your own preparation for your child's hospitalization
- Selecting the hospital

- How and when to change your child's doctor
- Participating in your child's hospital stay
- Emergency admissions
- Helping your child recover

Chapter **17**   LEAVING THE HOSPITAL   192

- Reviewing your bill
- Standard health insurance policies
- Major medical
- Medicare
- Medicaid

Chapter **18**   THE SOCIAL WORKER AS A MEMBER OF THE
HEALTH CARE TEAM AND A GUIDE TO
POSTHOSPITAL CARE   200

- Aiding the patient psychologically, financially,
  environmentally, and socially
- Community resources: visiting nurses, home
  health aid, therapists, and meals on wheels
- Equipment
- After-care facilities: rehabilitation centers,
  chronic disease hospitals, skilled nursing
  facilities, intermediate level nursing homes,
  domiciliary facilities, hospices, terminal care
  facilities

Index   207

To our wives, Barbara and Sandy,
for their patience, support, and
unfailing understanding

Introduction

The hospital—traditionally a place where the art of healing and the science of medicine clash headlong with the anxieties of the patient. Nobody likes to enter the hospital, even if it's going to make him better, and we all know why. Checking into a hospital means putting your total trust in strangers, in an alien place. For many people such dependency is frightening, it's almost a return to childhood. Added to that are the annoyances of patient life, unfamiliar procedures, and at times, a matter-of-factness on the part of the staff that may seem to you totally inappropriate.

Picture yourself recovering from a mild heart attack. Your program of relaxation includes blood pressure and temperature checks every four hours round-the-clock, the insufferable clatter of medication charts, housekeeping vehicles and food trays at all hours of the day and night, blood tests regularly at 5:00 A.M., and daily 7:00 A.M.. visits by an uninvited and unwelcome newspaper vendor. You can hardly wait to get home so that you can get the rest you need.

For those of you who have experienced irritating hospital moments, it may seem that hositals are "no place to be when you are sick." Sadly, in the past, hospitals perpetuated this attitude by too often overlooking the basic concerns of their VIPs, the patients themselves. Hospitals belong to you. They are there to serve you in times of need. But how successfully they do this depends a great deal upon how effectively you can make them work for you.

The hospital, in days past (fortunately new positive changes are in progress), encouraged blind compliance with frequently purposeless rules and regulations. Most people played the game: they were intimidated by the hospital scene. They meekly, unquestioningly accepted the problems they encountered and the nonsensical explanations for them. When a physician becomes a patient, he is rarely so tolerant. He knows what he wants and screams until he gets it; hence, the insiders' expression, "Doctors make lousy patients."

Somewhere between these extremes, of the timid patient and the overdemanding physician-patient, lies the "informed" patient. This patient understands how the system works and can manipulate it in a positive way. He or she can get the nurses "to bend the rules" for a good reason and still keep smiles on their faces. The informed patient may not be able to change basic routines or the sometimes impersonal attitude on the part of hospital staff, but he does understand what lies behind these annoyances and why, in some cases, they work ultimately to his advantage. He knows whom to call for help when a conflict arises, how effectively to lodge a complaint, and he does not confuse hostility with polite assertiveness. Helping the average person and his family to become successful hospital consumers is the goal of this book. We will reveal the inside workings of hospital life and offer many suggestions to help you use the hospital setting to your advantage, in the hope that such knowledge will make your hospital stay much more comfortable and far less frightening.

We have looked at patients' concerns from an unusual dual perspective. We are physicians; we understand many of the whys and wherefores of hospital shortcomings. At the same time we are deeply concerned with the needs of patients and the widening rift between the public and the medical system—a chasm that threatens to undermine the very fiber of patient care.

Our data come from many sources: the first was our personal experience in providing medical care ourselves (an early, if one-sided, view). Later we broadened our horizons by personally visiting, under the auspices of the Joint Commission on Accreditation of Hospitals, the Professional Standards Review Organization, and various other public and private organizations (including our own Quality Care Management Consultants), approximately fifteen hundred of the total seven thousand hospitals in the United States. These on-site visits, seminar programs, and teaching sessions enabled us to see and compare the inner workings of hospitals, ranging from the tiniest rural dispensary to the largest university facility. We met and conferred with scores of health care professionals and patients to probe the psychology, the concerns, the differences, and the common bonds that link both groups.

Together, we reviewed three thousand questionnaires that were given to patients in the hospital where one of us serves as director of Quality Assurance. These patient critiques and subsequent discussions with hundreds of the patients taught us a great deal—lessons that all doctors and nurses need to learn—about what makes patients tick and what makes their blood boil.

In this volume we are looking at the full range of medical care available in the United States and the broadest scope of surgical and medical crises that you may face. Ideally, your every problem, no matter how "minor or routine," should be managed in the world's greatest hospital. Obviously that is neither practical nor reasonable, and in fact, the majority of everyday health matters can be dealt with very well and very successfully in most medical centers—large or small, supersophisticated, or "just average." This, then, is not a plea to do away with your small-town hospital or a call for you to rush elsewhere for every ache or pain. It is an attempt to help you put your needs into proper focus, to compare those needs with the services that your hospital can effectively offer, and then to make intelligent decisions based upon realistic options.

It is also an attempt to share what we have learned about the inner workings of that strange world of hospitals, as only insiders can know it. With an informed background, you or your loved ones will be better prepared to take full advantage of the many services a modern hospital is now able to provide. From a calmer, less anxious perspective you will also be better able to smooth your way toward a rewarding recovery.

1

Why Choosing a Hospital Is One of the Most Important Decisions You May Ever Make

You are gazing out your kitchen window at the newly fallen snow. Suddenly the beauty and serenity of that picture is abruptly shattered. Your husband, who over your protests has been shoveling the walk and driveway for the past hour and a half, drops his shovel, clutches his chest, and falls to the ground. You rush to his side and find him ashen, his breathing labored, his brow covered with sweat. But he is alive and can at least speak haltingly.

By now the neighbors, alarmed by your cries, have called the fire rescue squad. In moments they arrive. A friend next door offers to look after the children. Still dazed, you whisper a worried thank-you and climb into the back of the rescue van with your husband and two attendants.

"We can go to either *Longview Community Hospital or the University Hospital. They're just about the same distance from here," offers one of the young men. "Do you have a preference? Maybe you have a personal physician who is on the staff of one."

---

* The name is fictitious. Any resemblance to a real hospital is accidental.

You tell them you really don't know, for although you do have a doctor, you haven't seen him for a while. You just can't think now, so you direct the attendants to do whatever they feel is best, to take him to the place where they'll give him the best care. Your voice cracks with emotion, your head swims with worries. How can you make a decision at a time like this?

"It looks like he's had a heart attack. They have a better coronary care unit at University Hospital, and they have physicians on duty there twenty-four hours. It's better for heart problems. We'll go there," volunteers one of them.

You look with gratitude and some sense of confidence at this man in his early twenties who is giving your husband some oxygen while his colleague places a needle into his vein and attaches a heart monitor. "They really seem to know what they're doing," you think. Your acute anxiety begins to fade. You are bolstered by their skill and good judgment.

It is touch and go for the first several days. Medicines continually flowing into his vein help the pumping of his heart and keep his blood pressure up. The administration of other drugs, at odd hours and at a moment's notice, stop his heart from beating erratically. After several days he stabilizes. His heart, over the acute crisis, regains some strength and begins to make it on its own. Two weeks later he is out of the coronary care unit and in an intermediate care section where he is still hooked up to various monitoring devices, but one-to-one nursing care is no longer needed. Instead, his vital functions are relayed to a nearby central station where one nurse can observe the television monitor of several patients. Two weeks more and he is on a regular floor, walking around, regaining his strength, preparing for his return home.

For a full month, the most harrowing time of both of your lives, University Hospital was home for your husband and home-away-from-home for you. Fortunately the paramedics chose the right hospital. If they hadn't, your husband might have died. You were asked to help them decide, but you couldn't. You knew less about your local hospitals than about the car you recently purchased. When you bought that new Oldsmobile, you painstakingly researched the alternatives. You read *Consumer Reports*. You spoke to friends. You compared performance ratings and specifications.

Then you knew which one was best, and you made your choice wisely. But when it came to "which hospital," far more important than "which car," you were caught off guard. You had not studied the local hospital scene. You had no idea what services each offered. So you left this life-and-death decision to strangers. They were available, competent, helpful, and correct. This isn't always the case.

The teak desk is piled high with journals, books, and patient charts. Across from you sits Dr. Thompson, family physician and confidant since you were a child thirty years ago.

"John, I've known you for a long time. I think we've built up a healthy respect for one another." He smiles, with what seems a somewhat strained expression. Though the words are kind and reassuring, your anxiety mounts.

"You know that cough you've been complaining about lately? There may be some explanation here in your chest X-ray. See this spot?"

He swivels around in his chair and flicks the switch on the X-ray view box. He doesn't have to point it out. On the right there is a large white patch, strikingly absent on the other side. Even you, an engineer with no medical training, can see that.

"Spot! It looks more like a cannonball!" you exclaim.

"It is fairly good sized, and it certainly needs some looking into. May be nothing at all, but it could be something serious. I'd like to refer you to Sam Turner; he's the surgeon in town. He'll want to run some special tests and probably put you in the hospital. It's even possible, depending on what the tests show, that he might need to operate."

The key words light up in your imagination like neon signs: *surgeon, hospital, operate.* Maybe it's cancer!" you think.

The rest of your discussion is a blur. You aren't sure whether you agreed to see Dr. Turner, or when and if you are going into the hospital. Several days pass; calm discussions with friends and your wife help you to focus your thoughts.

Sommerville is a town of only ten thousand people with a hospital so small it would probably fit inside the lobby of City Hospital, fifty miles west. As a layman you don't know the answer, but you intuitively feel that your problem could be serious and that Dr. Turner and Sommerville Hospital may not be the best place to be. You consult Dr. Thompson.

"John, our hospital is convenient for you and the family, although, I will admit, it isn't as well equipped as City Hospital. Turner is very good, but he doesn't specialize in chest problems. There isn't enough call for a full-time chest surgeon here in Sommerville. Assuming everything goes smoothly, as I'm sure it will, Sommerville Hospital and Dr. Turner will do well by you. But, if anything out of the ordinary comes up, I'll confess, you might be better off in City Hospital."

You feel misled and betrayed by your trusted physician. Angry thoughts arise, "Why didn't he tell me that before? How could he even suggest that I stay here when I can get better care in City Hospital? What if I hadn't asked?"

Dr. Thompson, noting your increasingly hostile expression, explains. "John, I suppose I should have given you the choice from the start. It's just that it rarely occurs to me. I believe in our medical care here. I don't think your problem is serious, at least I'm hoping and praying it's not, and I think Turner and Sommerville Hospital can do the job. But now and then I'm forced to remember that we aren't the top-of-the-line. Nothing to do with our commitment to our patients you understand. It's all a matter of size and economics."

The lanky physician looks uncomfortable, like a football player who has just admitted that his team is worse than the opponent's and then remembers his coach's dictum, "Never do that!" His uneasiness is heightened because you questioned his judgment, and were right. He now realizes that he should have given you the facts and let you decide from the start.

You are still annoyed, but you feel some empathy for the obviously embarrassed physician. "I want to go to City Hospital," you state without a second's hesitation. "Can you refer me to someone there?"

"As a matter of fact," says Thompson, "a classmate of mine from medical school is chief of the thoracic surgery section at City Hospital. Bill Steingold is an excellent chest surgeon and has a team of residents, interns, nurses, and fellows that have a fine reputation nationally. Would you like me to refer you to Bill?"

Bill Steingold was the perfect choice. In one week he had carried out a series of the most sophisticated tests available: bronchoscopy; tomography; cytological studies; special cultures for fungi, tuberculosis, and other infections; and a small biopsy of the spot, not by a serious operation but through a tube placed down your windpipe. The results are clear. No operation. No cancer. You have an infection that requires intensive treatment with special drugs, under the careful management of a specialist in infectious diseases. There is no such person in Sommerville, but City Hospital has one of the best. In less than a year the cough and the spot are completely gone.

"Why is it that kids always seem to get sick in the middle of the night?" you think to yourself as you fill out the emergency room form. Your three-year-old son, one thumb in his mouth, the other clutching his aching belly, is curled up in a waiting room chair.

"All the insurance information complete?" asks the gruff attendant, seemingly annoyed at being disturbed at 3:00 A.M.

"What else does she have to do anyway?" you think to yourself. "She works at night, doesn't she. She's getting paid to be here."

"Just sit and wait a while. I'll have to wake the doctor up. I'm not even sure where he is," she says disdainfully.

That last gratuitous comment seems like the final hint for you to go away. Your last chance to decide whether you *really* want to see the doctor or not. The moans of your son provide the answer. The child has to be seen by a doctor. You are, however, becoming increasingly sorry that you didn't call Dr. Cook, the pediatrician you chose when you recently came to town. You thought it would be easier, and certainly more convenient for Dr. Cook, if you took Billy right to the hospital. Perhaps you made a mistake.

Twenty minutes later the physician arrives. He is disheveled, young, and seemingly even more annoyed than the clerk at this unwelcome intrusion. He asks you curtly about your son's problem, but he doesn't seem to wait for the answer. He pokes at your child's swollen belly; Billy screams when he finds the tender spot on the right side. Then he says something quickly—the only word you can understand is "tests"—and he disappears.

The attendant returns to phone for the lab technician, appearing even more annoyed than she did on your first encounter. After a thirty-minute wait the technician arrives, disturbed at this interruption of his sleep and acting almost surly.

Until now you felt a bit cowed by the manner of the emergency room personnel. Maybe your son isn't that sick; you even find yourself hoping something really is wrong so you won't have put them to all this bother for nothing. Then suddenly you begin to feel furious at the way these people are dealing with other human beings—people for whose care they have accepted responsibility.

With all the finesse of a Mack truck, the laboratory technician inserts a needle four times before he finds Billy's vein and draws out some blood. He then instructs your screaming son to give him a urine specimen. Billy's in no mood, at this point, to cooperate.

Ninety minutes later the doctor returns. The laboratory studies are back. His examination, such as it was, is complete. "Your boy has appendicitis. He needs an operation. I'll call the surgeon," he announces.

You are stunned by this bombshell, but before you have a moment to regain some composure and ask some questions, he is out the door and on the phone.

"Wait a minute," you think to yourself. The mounting seriousness of the situation shakes you and sharpens your senses. "I don't like this place. I don't trust these people. I'm sure as hell not going to let my son have an operation here without talking to my husband and to Dr. Cook."

Your first call is to Dr. Cook. You tell him what has happened. He seems concerned and asks lots of questions about Billy: How much pain? Does he have a fever? When did the pain start?" And he doesn't seem annoyed at the nighttime intrusion. "Leave that hospital and meet me at Children's Hospital. It's only fifteen minutes away, and there are excellent surgeons and pediatric nurses there. He'll get better care. I'll see you shortly," he says reassuringly.

You cancel the call to the surgeon; inform your husband, who is at home with your other children; and make the drive to Children's Hospital.

Since you came to town only eight months ago, this was your initial hospital experience. The hospital you just left and Children's Hospital are as different as night and day. At Children's Hospital there are five or six children waiting to be seen; alert, considerate clerks; several physicians who seem to belong there and don't seem to mind the fact that it is nighttime; and two or three laboratory technicians who actually help soothe the children's jangled nerves.

Two minutes after you arrive Dr. Cook appears. He carefully examines your son from head to toe. He finds the same tender spot in the lower right of Billy's abdomen.

"The history and examination do suggest appendicitis," he counsels. "I want to repeat some of those blood tests and get some X-rays, but I am concerned enough to call in a surgeon while those tests are being done. Louis Samuels, an excellent surgeon, specializes in pediatric surgery. In fact, he recently operated on my daughter."

You are still concerned, but you now feel confident. This, you are sure, is the right place for Billy. You trust Dr. Cook and his judgment. If he recommends Dr. Samuels, that's good enough for you. With a sigh of relief you tell him, "Whatever you think, Doctor. I'll call my husband."

It was appendicitis. Dr. Samuels operated that night, well before the appendix burst. The pediatric nurses, who do nothing but take care of children, knew how to make Billy feel comfortable and at ease. The bright walls covered with Sesame Street characters and the presence of other children also helped a lot. In one week Billy was home. Later he occasionally talked about going back to visit all his friends. He remembered the hospital as the place where "big bird sleeped with me."

We'll return to the stricken snow shoveler, to John, and to Billy at the end of the chapter. We told their stories to illustrate an important point. When a trip to the hospital is inevitable you may have a choice: Which one? How well you choose may turn the tide for or against you. All hospitals are not alike.

Although the public is generally aware that there are differences in hospitals, few hospital "consumers" realize just how crucial and extreme those differences can be. To cite one example: many hospitals have no physicians on the premises at night. They depend on the availability of the private physician to handle the nurses' calls. That's fine as long as the patient isn't terribly sick and doesn't need moment-to-moment medical management, but for the critically ill patient, having to wait forty minutes for his doctor to get to the hospital can cost him his life.

A few years ago I worked in the emergency room of a small community hospital in southern California.* It was a friendly, pleasant environment: a good place to work, and a good place to be a patient if you weren't too sick. Unfortunately some of the patients were very sick. The hospital had a coronary care unit where heart attack victims, always touch and go in the first days after their attack, were placed. There they were watched by nurses who were well trained, to be sure, but not as qualified as a physician and not able to deliver the care that these patients deserved. The patients were hooked up to the latest monitors, which to their families was a sign of excellence. These devices made the relatives feel confident. In fact, these machines are guides to the patient's status. They help the nurses see what's going on. But when the heart rhythm suddenly changes, immediate physician action is needed. Lifesaving drugs must be ordered at once; emergency physician-controlled resuscitation may be mandatory.

There were several occasions when I received an urgent call at my emergency room post to assist a troubled patient in the coronary care unit. When I could, I went and did what was necessary until the private physician arrived. On at least three occasions I couldn't leave. I was in the midst of other lifesaving procedures with accident victims. I hoped that the heart patients had held out until help arrived, but I later learned that two of them did not survive the wait.

If this were in the middle of Alaska, the situation would be both understandable and unavoidable. There, medical care is in limited supply. Hospitals and patients make do with the best available help. But the hospital where I worked was approximately

---

* Although there are two authors, we use "I" throughout when presenting a personal experience.

thirty miles from downtown Los Angeles, in the midst of a metropolitan area of five million people. Exactly five miles down the road was the Orange County Medical Center, a fully equipped massive medical facility brimming with physicians day and night. Here, cardiologists or physicians finishing their specialty training in cardiology manned the coronary care unit round-the-clock. The emergency room was staffed by a separate group of emergency specialists whose sole hospital responsibilities were devoted to the patients who were brought there.

At my hospital the outer trappings were impressive. The machinery was modern; the television monitors gave the appearance of "the best of medical care." But a hospital that has machines without doctors is like a fire department packed with new trucks but no firemen. I suspect that if the families of those patients in the coronary care unit knew that their loved ones were in jeopardy when superb care was available right down the road, there would have been a community uproar.

Hospitals come in all sizes, shapes, and qualities. There are good ones, bad ones, large ones, and small ones, and most important of all, there are some well suited to perform certain functions but totally inadequate to handle others. As we move through the next few chapters, we will begin to understand why this is so and how you can tell whether or not a hospital is right for you. First, consider this question: What choice do you have?

The three patients we met in the beginning of this chapter give us some clues to the answer. The wife of the snow shoveler had two choices: Longview Community Hospital or University Hospital. She had never looked into the hospital situation in her neighborhood and, therefore, left it up to the paramedics. Fortunately, they chose wisely. They could just as easily have taken her husband to Longview where, like the southern California hospital, there were no physicians on duty at night. Her husband's precarious early days demanded fine-tuned management. Without doctors on the premises, he probably would have died.

John Billings had a choice. His problem was not urgent. He had a week or two to think it over. His family physician, Dr. Thompson, recommended the town hospital, but when John began to ask some questions, he confessed that City Hospital would be the better place. He was right. The lung problem was easily managed without an operation, but diagnosis required special expertise and highly sophisticated studies. If Dr. Turner, the one surgeon in town, had managed the case, John would likely have ended up with an unnecessary and dangerous operation, not because Dr. Turner is incompetent, but because he is less familiar with these special problems than Dr. Steingold at City Hospital.

Billy's mother could have agreed to the appendectomy at once. Instead she transferred her son to her own doctor at Children's Hospital. It is likely that the operation would have been successful in either place, but the chances were better at the Children's Hospital because specialists in children's diseases, including pediatricians and pediatric surgeons, took care of Billy. The nurses, too, were specialized. Their full-time professional involvement was in child care. Finally, Children's Hospital was a cheery place, a place which left Billy with happy memories of his hospital experience.

Obviously, for everyone in all situations, a choice of hospitals is not always possible. There are three factors which influence the choices you have: the urgency of the situation, the size of your community and the number of hospitals available, where your personal physician has staff privileges. Depending on your situation, any of these may determine where you *must* go—you may have no choice whatsoever—or else they may play a role in your decision but not present insurmountable obstacles.

If your automobile careens off the road while you are traveling in a strange state, leaving you unconscious and bleeding internally, you go to whatever hospital the ambulance takes you. If your husband collapses with a heart attack and there is only one hospital in town—the next nearest located thirty miles away—the town hospital is the place for him. But only in these cases of extreme emergency, when no other facilities are nearby, are your options so limited.

John lived in a small town with one hospital. When his problem, pressing but not life threatening, seemed too complex for Sommerville Hospital, he decided to go to the city, fifty miles away. Every state in this country has a top-notch medical center which is available and accessible to everyone. Sometimes the inconvenience of a fifty- or even two-hundred-mile trip is well worth it. A serious medical problem may call for a temporary move away from your small town.

Your doctor may want to admit you to the hospital down the road for a series of tests. Perhaps it's the only hospital where he has privileges. If you believe that your problem is too complicated for that hospital or if you have reason to believe, from friends' stories or from specific guidelines which our later chapters will give you, that the hospital is substandard, you owe it to yourself to consider going elsewhere. It may mean a temporary change of doctors, but if your physician is compassionate, he should understand your concerns.

We are not suggesting that the small hospital, the neighborhood hospital, the hospital with relatively limited facilities and personnel serve no purpose. In fact, the majority of most common medical and surgical problems can be handled quite efficiently there (except in the unusual case of the truly dreadful hospital— there are a few). To be a sophisticated consumer of hospital care you need to understand which problems are serious, which are not; which require special expertise, which do not; and when a hospital can or cannot serve you well. In the next two chapters we will try to help you evaluate your needs and the capabilities of your local medical facilities.

2

Assessing Your Needs

There are approximately seven thousand hospitals in the United States. They vary in size from sixty-bed infirmaries to mammoth three-thousand-bed inner-city complexes. It would be impossible for us to appraise each individually. In this and the following chapters we will offer some guidelines and general rules to follow and a number of special considerations to help you choose wisely. These standards and criteria should provide useful insights into the bewildering and too often awesome hospital world. These are the guidelines that we, as physicians, use in choosing a hospital for ourselves.

In the following pages when we refer to physicians, we may use "he," "she," or "he or she." Female physicians abound these days, but sometimes habit and common usage may make it seem as though we are favoring the men. We ask the women to forgive us.

When we talk about your "community" or "neighborhood" hospital, we are generally referring to smaller, less sophisticated facilities—the kind that might be found in a town of ten thousand, for example. For some of you this may seem confusing. For instance, if you live next door to Massachusetts General Hospital, your "neighborhood" hospital is both large and probably one of the best in the entire world. "Community," "local," "neighborhood" are simply terms that we find convenient in referring to less sophisticated (not necessarily bad) smaller hospitals. Big city residents may also have smaller, less sophisticated hospitals in their neighborhoods, but they have the added good fortune, generally, of having access to full-range facilities.

Keep in mind that you will not always have a choice of hospitals. Some of the reasons are obvious. A serious highway accident may send you to the nearest hospital. If you collapse at home with a stroke or heart attack, traveling the extra twenty minutes to reach the best hospital in town might be dangerous. If there are strong reasons to stay with your own physician and he or she is on the staff of only one hospital, that may be where you should go. If you live in a small isolated community with one hospital nearby, traveling one hundred miles to the closest large city may be neither feasible nor necessary. However, as we saw earlier, the trip may sometimes be worth it. As we move through this chapter, you should begin to understand when that may be the case.

The overall quality of a hospital is important, but much more relevant for you is its ability to take care of your special needs. Medical problems vary in complexity, from basic and routine to tremendously sophisticated. The very sophisticated hospital is best able to handle the entire range of these problems, but it is unnecessarily overtalented for everyday needs. For those, your local hospital is probably quite adequate. For the same reasons that you wouldn't buy a highway-sized snowplow to clear your twenty-foot driveway or hire Artur Rubinstein to give your five-year-old his first piano lessons, you do not need a major medical center for routine problems.

Most hospitals can handle standard surgery: D and Cs, hysterectomies, appendectomies, gallbladder operations, hernia repairs, cataract operations; minor diagnostic tests like X-rays of the kidneys and intestinal tract; wide varieties of blood studies; and straightforward medical problems like pneumonia, hepatitis, kidney infections, diabetic control. Unless your neighborhood hospital is abysmally poor, it can complement your doctor's care if you suffer from scores of conditions like these or require commonplace tests. At the same time it offers the pluses of familiarity, nearness to the comfort of friends and relatives, and care by your own physician. The small community hospital plays a vital role in our health care system.

How do you begin to assess your hospital needs? How do you know whether you need a "Cadillac," or whether a "Chevrolet" will do? If you have a personal physician who is competent, compassionate, someone you respect and can trust, begin with him or her. If you do not, you should find one. You may have to try out several before settling on the medical practitioner who best suits you. Many articles and books have been written on how to choose a physician. We refer you to your local library, to information available at the local medical societies, to recommendations from friends and neighbors. Examine your physician's credentials; consider the thoroughness with which he examines you; the time and care that he takes with your problems and concerns; and his willingness to accept polite, well-meaning questions. A physician who treats each question as another threat to his authority cannot help you in your search for proper hospital or medical care.

Even if you do have an excellent, kindly physician, you have the right and the duty to tactfully question his recommendations of hospitals and specialists. After all, he may be associated with only one or two, and even a well-meaning physician may find it hard to admit that his hospital or some of the specialists who practice there have deficiencies. Recall, for example, Dr. Thomas in Chapter 1. A concerned physician will understand your worries, respect your inquiries, and will work with you to make the proper choice. Once questioned by John, Dr. Thomas willingly referred him out of Sommerville to City Hospital.

The first considerations are: How serious a problem do you have? How dangerous are your scheduled tests or operation? Your doctor is the one to consult first for the answers.

There are also clues available to you. At the furthest extreme, common sense is your best guide. It doesn't take a medical education for you to realize that if you have just awakened after a massive heart attack and are hooked up to an arcade of machines in an intensive care unit, you need close observation and physician supervision. If your doctor tells you that you must undergo an open-heart operation, brain surgery, a kidney transplantation, you have a delicate, potentially difficult, road ahead. If you are in a catastrophic automobile crash that leads to major surgery and weeks of intensive care management, you must have superior management to pull through. If you awaken to find your mattress ablaze and subsequently learn that you have sustained burns to 60 percent of your body, your prognosis will depend on specialized burn care not available at most hospitals.

If your two-year-old child is found to have a major malformation of his digestive organs and requires complicated surgery, he won't survive unless he is cared for in one of the few dozen hospitals in the entire country that is geared to treat him. Problems and conditions like these obviously cry out for optimal, round-the-clock care in the most sophisticated setting available—one that has special expertise and daily practice in the management of these illnesses and injuries.

At the other extreme, some ailments are obviously trivial. Treatment for an infected toe, a sprained back, a small lump that can be taken out without putting you to sleep, or a minor but painful kidney stone will probably go smoothly wherever you are treated. Not that complications from even seemingly simple problems cannot occur. They can and do. Once in a few thousand times someone who started out with what appeared to be a minor problem may later regret having entered his small-town hospital. But life is full of chances, and as far as we are concerned, minor conditions that have a tiny chance of becoming major can be handled quite efficiently at most American hospitals.

Between these extremes of simple and treacherous conditions lie thousands of medical and surgical illnesses and scores of diagnostic procedures. Here is where you need some special medical insights—which we will try to provide—to get a clear understanding of your problem and the ability of your nearby hospital to handle it. At the end of this chapter we include a handy reference chart listing dozens of conditions and procedures and their relative complexities.

ROUTINE CARE: OUTPATIENT

If your care is too routine, you may not belong in a hospital. This is particularly important today when soaring health costs have led to increased vigilance by insurance companies. They won't pay your bill if a reviewer at the company does not believe that hospitalization was warranted. This means that routine tests are no longer grounds for hospitalization. Recently we encountered dozens of irate patients furious at their physicians and the hospital for putting them through a three-thousand-dollar hospital stay only to learn that Blue Cross wouldn't pay. Their anger mounted when they discovered that the same tests would have been paid for almost in full if they had been performed in the outpatient setting.

By now most physicians and most hospitals are aware of these insurance changes. But some may not be. Before you go into the hospital, be sure that the hospitalization is necessary: that the same procedures can't be handled with daily trips from home. Also be certain that all planned tests will be covered by your insurance. Ask your doctor. Ask the hospital admission clerk or cashier. It is sometimes wise to separate your tests into two groups: those that must be done in the hospital (requiring a few days' stay) and those that can be handled in a clinic on an outpatient basis.

ROUTINE CARE: HOSPITAL

In general, operations that can be done under local anesthesia or ones which may require only a few minutes of general anesthesia (where you are put to sleep) are not likely to demand the most sophisticated hospital care. These may include cataract surgery, tubal ligations, abortions, D and Cs, rectal and stomach biopsies performed through a scope rather than through an operation, ear operations, draining of abscesses under the skin, minor skin grafting, and operations on the hands and feet. The skill of the surgeon is still important, and the result may be directly related to his or her surgical expertise. But assuming you have found a qualified surgical specialist, most reasonably equipped and reasonably staffed hospitals can effectively and safely manage these conditions. There are very few catastrophes to worry about. You will not require eagle-eye supervision. A visit by a nurse once every four hours and daily doctor visits will probably suffice.

There are many nonsurgical conditions that may be best treated in a hospital, but are not life threatening. You step on a nail, and develop a badly infected leg that requires antibiotic injections. You should have nurses looking in on you periodically, but you are not likely to need immediate physician attention in the middle of the night. Or you may be a diabetic and have had difficulty regulating your insulin dosage. Your doctor may want you in the hospital to have the nurses help get you on track: a straightforward problem that is not likely to erupt into a serious emergency. Perhaps your blood pressure is very high, and your doctor wants you to have some "routine" tests, and trials of various medications. Most hospitals are well equipped to deal with this.

Many tests are quite routine. Your doctor may want you in the hospital to check out your unusual tiredness, bouts of stomach pain, joint aches, or trouble with your bowel movements. For these you may need a variety of blood tests; urine tests; ordinary X-rays; or slightly more complicated X-rays, such as special kidney X-rays (intravenous pyelogram), X-rays of your stomach and intestines (upper and lower gastrointestinal X-rays—barium swallows and barium enemas), or X-rays of your gallbladder (oral cholecystogram). Although many of these can be done on an outpatient basis, your doctor may prefer you to be in the hospital. Most hospitals can carry out these studies efficiently and accurately.

Routine hospital care, as the name implies, means "nothing extraordinary." If you require routine care, whether you live in a small rural community served by a modest hospital, a suburban area housing several middle-sized hospitals, or in the center of a large city where a massive university medical center is just around the corner, your health needs can be handled locally. Unless new problems are uncovered or unexpected difficulties arise, your neighborhood hospital, large or small, can help you.

❧

SECOND-LEVEL SURGICAL CARE

"Second-level care" is a term we constructed for problems that go beyond the routine but can be dealt with efficiently at many medium-sized, reasonably well equipped and well staffed hospitals. These are conditions and procedures that require some special expertise by nursing and medical staff. They require skilled implementation and moderately close observation. At the same time they are not extraordinary or supersophisticated.

The majority of everyday operations that require general anesthesia and close postoperative attendance fall into this group. Gallbladder operations, stomach operations, thyroid surgery, minor blood vessel operations, amputations, bowel surgery, ulcer operations, appendectomies, and hernia operations are a few common examples. How well you come through these operations depends upon several factors: how sick you are and how extensive an operation is required, your general health and age, the quality of the surgeon, the quality of the anesthetist, and the quality and abundance of nurses to care for your immediate postoperative needs. The first two are beyond your control. The last three are part of the hospital scene and should be examined as you evaluate the hospital.

How to Protect Yourself From the Most Dangerous Aspect of Surgery

Nonphysicians are generally surprised to learn that the most dangerous aspect of an operation in which you are put to sleep is not the operation itself. It is the anesthesia. It is the anesthetist, much more than your surgeon, who has control of your vital functions. (The term *anesthetist* refers in general to the person administering anesthesia. This may be either a physician, usually called an anesthesiologist, or a nurse, usually called an anesthetist, who is a specially trained registered nurse.) No matter how minor an operative procedure may be, if you are asleep, you place your life in the hands of that anesthetist. He or she must be certain every second that adequate oxygen is getting into your lungs and that your heart is pumping effectively. On occasion, fortunately relatively rare, individuals who undergo minor operations die during the procedure, not because of a surgical error, but from a problem related to the anesthesia.

The caliber of anesthesia practice in this country is more variable, and often lower, than the quality of surgical practice. The reason: there are not enough trained anesthesiologists to go around. They are supplemented by general physicians, not specifically trained in anesthesiology, and by nurse anesthetists, who are registered nurses with special training in anesthesia management. It would be ideal if all anesthesia could be administered by physicians with advanced training in anesthesiology. Unfortunately the limited supply precludes this. For the same reason, it is impractical for you to insist that a level-two procedure be managed entirely by a board-certified anesthesiologist. If that can be done, great! If not, there are certain safety checks you can make.

You're probably wondering, "Isn't that the surgeon's job? Why do I have to get involved with this? Won't he choose the best one for me?" Unfortunately, your surgeon may not participate in the choice, either because that isn't the way it's done at his hospital or because there simply isn't much choice. Therefore, since it's your operation and your life, you owe it to yourself to inquire and participate.

In most cases your anesthetist is assigned by the anesthesia department, either the night before or on the morning of your operation. The surgeon has nothing to do with the choice of anesthesiologists or nurse anesthetists. Occasionally certain surgeons, particularly those with some clout at the hospital, may have one or two favorite anesthetists and may request or insist that one of them do the job. Or, conversely, the surgeon may think that a certain anesthetist poses a real danger to his patients and will refuse to operate with him or her. You'd be amazed to learn how common this is! But most often the surgeon does not participate in the choice. And, as we've indicated above, in many places the choices are rather limited anyway. For example, in some isolated small hospitals there may be one or two individuals who administer anesthesia and whose performance ranges in quality from fair to very poor.

Your best bet is to resolve the anesthesia question before you even enter the hospital. You may not be able to pick the actual person beforehand, but you can attempt to assess the overall quality of anesthesia management at the hospital where you intend to go. Talk with your surgeon in his office. Let him know that you are concerned about the anesthesia, and are aware that expert handling of this phase of your operation is crucial. Ask whether a fully trained anesthesiologist, a resident physician training in anesthesiology, an untrained physician anesthesiologist, or a nurse anesthetist will be putting you to sleep and keeping a watchful eye on you throughout the procedure. If it is going to be an anesthesiologist, ask him whether the individual will be either board certified or a closely supervised resident and whether he will be a highly regarded member of the surgical team. Ask him to participate in the choice, to help you get the individual he would want for his own operation. If he seems hesitant or unduly defensive when you discuss these concerns with him, you should find out why. Perhaps the only person giving anesthesia in that fifty-bed hospital is a semiretired seventy-five-year-old general practitioner who is known to fall asleep during operations. Believe it or not, there are places that have abysmally poor anesthesia practices like this. You should know what you're in for before you agree to be put to sleep.

You may learn that the hospital uses nurse anesthetists. Many are competent and experienced and can give anesthesia very safely. They should, however (except in the most remote areas), be supervised closely by an anesthesiologist, preferably one who is board certified. If your anesthesia will be given by a nurse, ask whether a trained anesthesiologist is standing by—not on call at another hospital ten miles away as some are—in the event of a problem. Before you can proceed with confidence, you need a "yes" answer to this question. You should also inquire about the training, experience, and reputation of the nurse anesthetist. You would certainly not want be put to sleep by an individual who has encountered ten unexpected deaths and an equal number of malpractice suits in the past few years.

If your surgeon cannot answer your questions about the

anesthesia care in a manner that is fully satisfying, you have a decision to make: take your chances or go somewhere else. Your decision must depend upon a number of factors: how bad the anesthesia situation sounds; how serious your operation is and how long you'll have to be asleep; how close you are to another better-staffed hospital; how urgent your situation is; and whether you are willing, if necessary, to change surgeons for the sake of better anesthesia.

Most level-two procedures are not so urgent that a move to another hospital is impossible. An exception might be a planned appendectomy if the move could cause a several hour or more delay. If you live in a metropolitan area and you find that your neighborhood hospital has no anesthesiologist in attendance, you might consider a move elsewhere. Whether or not you choose to make that move depends upon your relationship with the surgeon and how strongly you want him to do the operation; a move may mean changing surgeons. Finally, if your are in a small, isolated community, it may not be worth the hundred-mile commute to the nearest large hospital. If your hospital is staffed by competent, experienced, well-regarded nurse anesthetists, the chances are that the procedure will go smoothly. You should be aware, however, that there is some added risk of having general anesthesia without having an anesthesiologist close by. That risk may be slight and may, for you, be worth taking.

How to Judge the Competence of Your Surgeon

Assessing the quality of the surgeon obviously is important. Many operations are still being done by general practitioners with little or no special surgical training. Except in the most remote areas and under the most urgent of circumstances, you should be certain that your surgeon has special training in surgery. He or she should have completed a residency and should be either board certified or board eligible. Ask him if he is. Look for the certificates on his wall. Also ask him how many operations of your type he has performed in the past two or three years, or in his entire career. If a surgeon is generally qualified but is in totally unfamiliar territory in your case, you will probably want to find someone else.

If you are reluctant to ask the surgeon himself about his training and experience in his specialty, ask your medical doctor. Presumably, if your case is typical, he referred you to him. You can also ask the local county or state medical society to give you some background information, including amount of training, where he trained, and whether or not he has been certified or deemed eligible by his specialty board. *(Board eligible* refers to someone who has completed training in a certified residency program but has not yet taken, or passed, a specialty-board examination. *Board certified* refers to one who is not only fully trained but has also passed his specialty-board examination.) Board eligibility or certification is no guarantee of excellence, but it is one guideline. At least it tells you that you are entrusting your life to someone who has some specialized, advanced training.

Other Factors Influencing the Outcome of Your Surgery

Finally, the outcome of your operation can be influenced by the quality and quantity of nursing care afterwards. You want to be certain that the hospital has a well-equipped, well-staffed recovery room, with nurses particularly experienced in postoperative care. You want to be in a place that has adequate surgical nursing care on the floor where you will reside for the one- to two-week convalescent period. Preferably this should be a section of the hospital set aside for postsurgical care. That gives you the best assurance that the nurses there will be attuned to your special needs. Speak with your doctor, any friends who have been in the same hospital, and anyone on the hospital staff whom you know in order to glean some insight into the quality of nursing care. In the next chapter we will offer additional guidelines to help you with this assessment.

For most second-level surgical problems emergency physician care is not needed in the postoperative phase. Exceptions exist. The very elderly patient, the individual who was quite sick prior to the operation, the person who develops a serious postoperative complication, may need instant physician intervention. But for the otherwise young, healthy individual, once the operation is over, the acute hazards have passed. Complications which may occur later generally arise gradually and can be picked up with routine nursing observation and a daily visit by the operating surgeon or the general medical practitioner. Consequently, if your planned operation is relatively minor, and if you are in good health generally, you can receive adequate care in a hospital where physicians are not on the premises at night—assuming, of course, that the nurses are attentive and your physician is available and a short distance away.

SECOND-LEVEL MEDICAL PROBLEMS

Second level medical problems (as opposed to second-level surgical problems) are a different matter. In these we include medical emergencies—strokes, heart attacks, seizures, severe asthma—and severe infections—meningitis or serious pneumonias. Most hospitals take patients with these conditions. Not all are well equipped to properly handle them. In Chapter 1 we gave some examples of serious deficiencies. Unless a qualified physician is in the hospital at all times, ready to take emergency action in case of patient deterioration or acute change, hospital care is seriously deficient.

At the risk of being repetitious, we must reiterate: your control of the situation may vary, depending upon the nature of your community, the services generally available, and the urgency of the clinical condition. However, if you have any choice—if there are several hospitals to choose from, if you can control where the ambulance takes you, or if transfer is possible—be sure that touch-and-go medical problems like these are managed in a place where a qualified physician is no more than moments away.

How to Find Out About a Hospital—and When to Do It

Take the following steps before the crisis arises. Ask the administrator of the local hospital or your doctor these questions: Who covers medical emergencies at night? Is there a physician *in the hospital* at night who watches the coronary care unit and the intensive care unit? Is he someone in addition to the emergency room physician, or is there only one person for both? What are the qualifications of the night physician? Is he specialty trained, or is he an unlicensed foreign medical graduate? This is not to imply that foreign physicians are necessarily bad. If their training, particularly their specialty training, is good, they may be fine physicians. Many hospitals, however, use newcomers who are relatively inexperienced, possibly fresh out of medical school, and not even licensed to practice medicine in the United States. Be wary of hospitals that staff their critical care units with these unskilled physicians.

Your hospital stay may involve special procedures or tests. As we saw earlier, some of these are routine and well handled anywhere. Others are more sophisticated—what we would call second-level procedures: myelography, a study of the spinal cord in which dye is injected into the spinal canal and X-ray pictures are taken; pneumoencephalography, an air study of the brain; bronchography, a special X-ray of the tubes leading to the lungs; arteriography, dye studies of various arterial systems, particularly the legs and kidneys, are some examples. Other forms of arteriography, including studies of the brain vessels, the heart, the coronary arteries, are even more specialized in terms of the expertise needed to carry them out and the potential complications that can occur. These we would classify as "level-three procedures."

Level-two procedures can be done competently in many moderately sophisticated hospitals. The requirements are a specialized staff of medical experts (generally radiologists particularly trained or experienced with these procedures or surgical specialists, such as neurosurgeons or vascular surgeons, with equally advanced training or expertise) and a staff of X-ray technicians well versed in these studies. The hospital that gives one such test every few months is not the best place to have it done. Repetition and experience are needed for quality performance and interpretation of these tests. Find out the following from whoever is recommending one of these tests to you: Who will be doing it? What special expertise does he or she have? How many of these do they do a week? Is there another hospital in town where the procedure can be performed more expertly?

❦

THIRD-LEVEL SURGICAL CARE AND PROCEDURES

There are some operations and certain studies that should only be carried out in highly skilled hospital settings. Most university hospitals—those associated with a medical school—would qualify. Some large medical centers, well staffed by a full range of medical and surgical specialists, can also serve these functions. These are tests and procedures that cannot be taken lightly. If you need one, you owe it to yourself to research the hospital before you go.

All brain, spinal cord, and heart operations fall into this category. Certain other sophisticated operations like kidney transplantation, major lung operations, and major vascular operations are other examples. It should be self-evident that these are extremely complex procedures. They involve vital organs that if damaged or compromised by the surgery can cause death or serious injury. The best of specialized surgical care by board-certified neurosurgeons, vascular surgeons, and cardiac surgeons is the first requirement. Top-notch anesthesia by fully trained anesthesiologists is mandatory. Superb postoperative nursing care by specially trained nurses is a must. A full-time, night-and-day staff of skilled medical personnel is essential.

Thus, all the elements that we discussed earlier as hallmarks of a Cadillac hospital must be present before you agree to one of these procedures. These elements are so important to the outcome that, except in the most dire of emergencies, you should not let distance stand in your way. If you have to travel to another state to find the best hospital available, make the trip.

The fact that the hospital simply does these operations does not mean it is the place to be. For example, there are large cities in which ten hospitals can do open-heart surgery. All are staffed by cardiac surgeons. But in most cases only one or two of them are doing a large volume—the amount needed to keep the surgical team fine tuned. If we had the choice of having our hearts operated on by a surgeon who does three cardiac cases a month, in a hospital that dusts off the heart-lung equipment when an operation is scheduled, or going to the neighboring place where the cardiac team operates every day, we would choose the latter. Practice and frequency are critical in maintaining high quality.

There are certain highly specialized tests or procedures which also fall into this category. They require special expertise and daily practice. Cardiac catheterization, where dye is injected into the heart to examine heart function; coronary artery catheterization, to look for narrowing of the blood vessels that feed the heart; cerebral arteriography, to evaluate the blood vessels of the brain; pulmonary arteriography, to check for blockage of the arteries entering the lungs; and specialized body scans, such as CAT (computerized axial tomography) scans, that use computers and special X-ray techniques to look for abnormalities in various parts of the body all demand special handling. Ideally they should be performed by radiologists with subspecialty training in these fields. Occasionally some of these, like pulmonary arteriography and CAT scans, may be done for emergency diagnosis. In those cases a choice of hospitals may be impossible.

༄

THIRD-LEVEL MEDICAL CARE

Certain medical problems fall into the category of "third-level illnesses." Many of these initially have the outward appearance of less serious conditions, but as time passes the picture changes. Consider this example: you are hospitalized in your community hospital because of some recent problems with tiredness, weakness, weight loss, and a few blackout spells. After several weeks of exhaustive testing your problem remains undiagnosed. There are some general internal medicine specialists about who have seen you briefly and come up empty-handed. Your family physician is baffled and is ready to throw his hands up and send you home no closer to a solution than when you entered the hospital. Needless to say, you are distraught and dissatisfied.

Make no mistake. Even the best medical minds and the

fanciest diagnostic testing cannot always come up with a satisfactory answer. Medicine is not that perfect. But before you go home and resign yourself to the life of an invalid, you owe it to yourself and your family to be absolutely sure that the best medical opinions and the best testing were utilized in your evaluation. You may require third-level evaluation in a top-notch medical center. There you will find even more specialized physicians, such as endocrinologists, rheumatologists, hematologists, and the diagnostic tools that offer the best hope for a diagnosis. A tactful request to your physician for a referral to such a center may be in your best interest.

Or perhaps you have a complicated and difficult-to-manage illness. You have spent the past three weeks in your local hospital under the care of your private physician and the available specialists in your community. Your disorder—diabetes, pituitary gland dysfunction, rheumatoid arthritis, to give a few examples—just does not seem to be responding well to the therapy. You may need the most specialized care available. There are physicians who devote all of their attention to a specific illness. They are the superspecialists. This term does not necessarily imply that they are overall better than any other specialist, but it does imply very specialized knowledge and expertise in a particular disease. For instance, there are physicians who specialize in diabetes, gout, rheumatoid arthritis, cancers, leukemia, infectious diseases. Perhaps you need an evaluation and management by one of these experts. Third-level care at a university or other major medical center may be in order. Ask your physician to refer you there.

SPECIAL CARE NEEDS

Certain individuals, either because of their age or the nature of their medical problems, may find that their local hospital simply cannot offer the right care for them. The specialized equipment and personnel necessary to treat pediatric or childhood diseases, as well as physical therapy, rehabilitation, and long-term chronic care, are "special needs" that not all hospitals can provide.

We all know that emotionally, intellectually, and socially children are not merely miniature adults. They are small, but they are also different. The same holds true for their illnesses and medical needs. Children get different illnesses from those of adults, and they respond in unique ways. Doctors and nurses who care for children must, therefore, be familiar with these distinctive little people.

If the child is not terribly sick, most experienced family physicians and certainly most pediatricians can do a capable job of handling his needs. However, just as with the adult, as the problem becomes more complex, "ordinary or average care" may not be good enough. Moreover, although the local hospital may be equipped to handle level-two adult illnesses, its nurses and physician staff may be unattuned to the needs and the special care of sick children. One of us had a recent experience which graphically illustrates this point.

One evening a frantic call came from a relative who lived approximately thirty miles from a major northeastern city. Her eight-month-old child had fallen down the basement steps and smashed his head against the concrete. We asked some of the proper questions by phone: Is he alert? crying? vomiting? sitting normally? It is, however, impossible to correctly diagnose and treat by phone. In addition, though my wife and I are both physicians, neither of us is expert in pediatric head trauma. Family members, of course, have implicit faith that their physician relatives are blessed with a full breadth of medical knowledge. Even though that is not the case, we are always flattered by this familial confidence.

In one sense, and one sense only, their confidence is justified. We do know where to go for help. We suggested that the child be taken to the children's hospital in town, one of the best in the country. The drive was about forty miles, but we felt the extra measure of reassurance would be worth it. On the staff of the hospital there are, of course, pediatricians, but there are also pediatric radiologists who are particularly adept at taking and reading children's X-rays, X-ray technicians who spend all of their working hours keeping children still for the pictures, and neurologists and neurosurgeons who specialize in children and, therefore, can pick up subtle abnormalities much more quickly than the specialist who sees mostly adults.

Our advice was rejected, and the mother took the child to the local family pediatrician who examined the child and ordered X-rays. They were taken at their small community hospital where they were interpreted as normal. We were not hurt or overly alarmed by this decision. The child did not, after all, appear to have suffered a serious injury.

Two days later the picture changed. The child's head began to swell massively, and a line showed up in his temple area. Another call to us raised our concern. Even our limited expertise brought forth the image of a fractured skull—internal bleeding—a potentially serious problem, one that might require surgery. The local pediatrician minimized the new finding and seemed to write it off as mostly maternal hysteria, but the graphic description by several nonmedical but observant family members convinced us otherwise. We again suggested a trip to the children's hospital. The mother came up with an alternative plan. How about reviewing the X-rays with the radiologists at the original hospital; taking new ones focusing on the exact site of the swelling; and then if a fracture showed up, transferring the child downtown. Okay, we would stay by the phone to monitor the progress and, perhaps, talk to the doctors. The events that followed shocked us and made it crystal clear that the child was in the wrong hospital and that a change of pediatricians should be the next order of business for this family.

They brought the child to the hospital; the pediatrician had agreed with this. Then they asked to speak to the radiologist. Apparently at that hospital radiologists do not talk to people. They look at pictures and talk to dictating machines. The radiologist grabbed the original X-rays, stormed out annoyed that the parents would even presume to ask for a moment of his time, and immediately informed their pediatrician of their arrogance. The phone rang in the X-ray suite. It was a call to the mother from the family pediatrician, "How dare you ask to speak to the radiologist! Who the hell do you think you are?" With that they properly grabbed their child and made the drive to Children's Hospital.

There the atmosphere and the approach were entirely different. First there was a complete exam by a pediatrician, then a consultation and examination by the neurosurgeon. Finally the radiologists saw the child, pinpointed the area that needed to be X-rayed, and ordered proper films. What they revealed was a fracture! The child's skull was indeed broken. Fortunately the story has a happy ending. The child's brain was, apparently, uninjured. The fracture is healing. And the baby is being following closely by the children's hospital specialists. But we all shudder to think of what might have happened had the possible dire consequences of intracranial bleeding ever materialized.

There is a twofold lesson in this story. It tells us about unfeeling physicians who do not respond sympathetically to patients' needs or concerns. Another pediatrician would probably have referred the child to the children's hospital, recognizing that this was a special problem requiring special expertise. At the very least, he would have asked for help from the radiologist and worked with him to X-ray the danger spot. The story also shows you that children are different. X-rays are more difficult to read. Positioning is crucial. What may appear normal to the radiologist who sees very few children's films in his daily practice, may stand out boldly as a fracture to a reviewer more familiar with this situation.

Thus, if you are not satisfied with the care your child receives, if you are dissatisfied with the answers you get or with the examination that is performed, if your child is hospitalized on a ward occupied mostly by adults, you should be asking these questions: Is this the best place? Are the physicians and nurses here in touch with the unique needs and problems that children face? If not, would another hospital, either one which deals solely with children or one with a large pediatric practice, be better?

There are other special care needs that not all hospitals can handle. If your grandmother has a hip fracture and faces replacement of her natural bone by a metal joint, her recovery depends upon much more than the operation itself. The same is true if an amputation is the intended procedure. Certainly the orthopedic surgeon should be skilled to ensure the best surgical outcome. Beyond that, your grandmother will have to go to a special school to learn how to walk again. That school—a hospital's physical therapy department—does just as much as the surgeon to help get her back on her feet and back to a useful life. A hospital that does not have a full-range physical therapy department staffed by trained therapists and, preferably, run by a physician therapist cannot provide the best postoperative care. Consider then the full scope of an illness—both the immediate and long-range needs. Inquire. Can the hospital do a good job with both? If not, there may be another nearby that can. Since patients who need a hip replacement or an amputation may not be in dire straits, a transfer or admission elsewhere may be feasible.

LEVELS OF CARE: CAN YOUR HOSPITAL SATISFY YOUR NEEDS?

	STUDIES	MEDICAL	SURGICAL
Routine	· Blood test · Urine test · Upper GI X-ray · Lower GI X-ray · Intravenous pyelogram (kidney X-ray) · Cholecystogram (gallbladder X-ray) · Simple X-rays—chest, bones	· Minor infection · Routine diabetic control (not for patient in coma) · Kidney stone (no operation) · Evaluation of various conditions—high blood pressure, anemia, tiredness	Many of the operations can be done with either local or general anesthesia. They fall into "routine" if done with local anesthesia. Some examples: · Cataract (with local) · Tubal ligation · D and C · Abortion · Minor biopsies · Ear surgery · Skin grafting · Minor hand and foot surgery · Hemorrhoid surgery (with local) · Traction
Second Level	· Myelography (spinal cord X-ray) · Pneumonencephalography · Bronchography · Some arteriography · Bone marrow studies · Kidney, liver, or other closed biopsies · Scans—liver, spleen, bone, thyroid, brain, etc.	· Stroke · Heart attack · Severe seizure · Severe asthma · Serious infection	· All operations needing general anesthesia · Operations needing spinal anesthesia · Stomach surgery · Thyroid surgery · Most blood vessel surgery · Mastectomy · Amputation · Bowel Surgery · Hernia operation

LEVELS OF CARE: CAN YOUR HOSPITAL SATISFY YOUR NEEDS?

	STUDIES	MEDICAL	SURGICAL
			· Appendectomy · Ulcer surgery · Laminectomy · Pacemaker insertion · Hysterectomy
Third Level	· Cardiac catheterization · Coronary artery catheterization · CAT scan (computerized axial tomography) ** · Pulmonary arteriography	· Complex disorders *— difficult to diagnose or difficult to manage · Seriously ill newborns	· Brain surgery * · Spinal cord surgery · Kidney transplantation · Major lung operation · Major blood vessel surgery · Open-heart surgery · Coronary artery bypass surgery · Severe burns · Major trauma

* Levels are graded either according to the dangers of the procedures; or the ** special expertise needed to do them and evaluate them properly.

3

Which Hospital Is Best for Your Needs

We have seen that illnesses and health care needs are as diverse and individual as people themselves. A hospital that is perfect for certain services may be dreadful for others. One may ensure a smooth recovery; another may invite tragedy. The wise hospital consumer understands what determines quality hospital care.

Let us substitute the term "sophisticated" for "quality," for many unsophisticated rural hospitals deliver high quality care. They simply cannot provide the range of services and the breadth of expertise of their more extensive counterparts. Thus, no perjorative is implied when we rate certain hospitals above others. A hospital may be very good at what it does. It may handle routine matters superbly, but it may lack the resources and capabilites of the larger center.

We have used the terms "larger" and " smaller" a number of times, almost interchangeably, with "sophisticated" and "un-sophisticated." To some extent this is an oversimplification, but for the most part, it holds true. Communities that can support a very large hospital—six hundred beds or more—can also support a full complement of medical and surgical specialists and a wide range of diagnostic capabilities. This gives us one usual hallmark of sophistication—size. Larger hospitals are generally more sophisticated than small ones. There are obviously exceptions. A massive, three-thousand-bed inner-city hospital may be in utter decay, its facilities abysmal, because of the loss of city financial support. Or a highly affluent suburban community may be blessed with an overabundance of superspecialist physicians who work out of the neighborhood's two-hundred-bed hospital. If one of these situations exists near you, you are probably aware of it. The small neighborhood hospital has a well-deserved reputation for excellence and sophistication. The ramshackle city hospital is a place you wouldn't want to go to even for a stubbed toe.

What makes one hospital better or more sophisticated than another? The quality and breadth of its medical staff; the ready availability of physicians in the hospital; the most complete range of diagnostic equipment and treatment facilities; and top-notch nurses who are not so overworked that they cannot pay proper attention to each patient.

҈

UNIVERSITY HOSPITALS

There is a standing joke among doctors: show the academic physician a patient with meningitis, lupus erythematosus, pituitary gland dysfunction, a liver tumor, or dengue fever and his heart will flutter with excitement. But a child with chickenpox, or someone with a cold or simple appendicitis—forget it. He'll either be out of his element or he won't care. As with most clichés, this one is laced with a few elements of truth.

University hospitals are centers of higher education and frontiers of medical progress. Challenging, esoteric illnesses feed the imagination and stimulate the creative scholarly instincts of academic physicians. Mundane, run-of-the-mill illnesses do not. Thus, the patient with a stone-filled gallbladder, a mild asthmatic attack, or a migraine headache may not be the subject of exciting discussions on morning rounds. But that doesn't mean that these patients won't get excellent care. The university hospital offers a broad, full range of medical capabilities.

The university hospital is geared to evaluate and care for patients with most medical and surgical diseases. And, in general, it is equipped and staffed to do the job ably. Within its walls is a complement of general physicians—internists, obstetricians, pediatricians, surgeons. What's more, unlike less sophisticated hospitals, it has a staff of superspecialized subspecialists who limit their practice to certain organs or certain diseases. There are liver specialists, experts in infectious diseases, cancer specialists, diabetologists, chest surgeons, vascular surgeons, and many more.

In general, university-based physicians or those with active university affiliations are at the forefront of new medical happenings. Because they are usually teaching, they remain attuned to recent developments in broad ranges of medical and surgical problems. Hence, both the generalists and the superspecialists at the university medical centers can offer the most sophisticated, most current diagnostic and therapeutic approaches to your problems. If your condition is highly complex, or technically difficult, a university hospital is often the best place to be.

The university hospital nurses too are generally well attuned to the problems of their patients. Because they constantly face the probes and questions of a medical team and must answer to physicians daily, they are forced to keep good records and make careful observations. They are an important part of a smoothly functioning unit. They know it, and they generally respond appropriately. There is a certain pride that nurses at the finer university hospitals feel. Just as the physicians are proud to say they are associated with Harvard, Johns Hopkins, the University of Michigan, the University of Pennsylvania, the University of California, Vanderbilt, Yale, or Columbia, nurses too feel the same pride in these institutions. These places (and many others that are not mentioned) attract nurses who enjoy the personal satisfaction of being a part of "the best."

University hospitals are, overall, at the pinnacle of medical excellence. However, just as universities themselves vary in quality, so do their affiliated hospitals. Some may be stronger in certain specialties and disciplines than others. A few may actually be worse than an excellent nonuniversity hospital—even one in the same city. The quality of the university hospital is determined by the quality of the medical staff it attracts. This, in turn, is dependent

upon the financial resources of the institution and their commitment to academic superiority. In general, the quality of the medical center parallels the quality of the university with which it is
affiliated. Thus, if you know universities and their reputations, you
have some notion about their medical schools and their university
hospitals.

Other Teaching Hospitals

A teaching hospital is any hospital that has students, either
medical students, postgraduate physicians-in-training, fellows, or
all of these. There are many fine teaching institutions that are
closely affiliated with medical schools but are not the primary
university hospital. These may have all of the desirable characteris-
tics noted in the discussion above, particularly if the university
with which it is affiliated is first-rate. Others may have no medical
school ties and yet have an excellent staff and a full complement of
qualified postgraduate training physicians. A prime example was
the Mayo Clinic. A fine medical center, the Mayo Clinic now has
its own medical school, but until a few years ago, it did not. It had
residents and fellows, but it was not a university hospital. Yet the
breadth of excellent specialty care and sophistication was, and still
is, outstanding. The Washington Hospital Center in Washington
D.C., is another example. It is a private institution with no major
medical school ties. Yet it has good postgraduate training programs and a wide range of medical services and specialists.

How and When to Find the Best Teaching Hospital

If you have a particularly delicate, very esoteric, or highly
specialized medical problem, good or even very good may not be
good enough for you. If I had a brain tumor, for example, I would
not be satisfied with the nearest neurosurgeon, even if he were
associated with university hospital. I would (if there were time, of
course) research him and the hospital before having my skull
opened. I would assure myself that the surgeon was well respected

and well qualified and that he, the hospital, and the anesthesiologists were performing enough of these procedures—several per month at least—so that they had sufficient practice. If this were not the case, I would ask for a referral to the surgeon and center in the country where they were most expert in that particular operation. One way for the more adventuresome and research-inclined individual to find such information is to review medical literature. Standard textbooks in the particular field and current medical writings are available at all medical libraries. All medical schools, for example, have them. You can look up your particular problem and find out who is studying it and writing about it most actively. Please understand, this does not apply to common disorders. It is not necessary to take your inflamed appendix, your cataract, your stone-filled gallbladder, your stomach ulcer, or your hernia to the finest medical center or greatest authority in the world. Any reasonably capable, well-trained surgeon can handle those. We are talking about unusual, highly delicate, complex procedures that fall outside the realm of average daily practice in the community hospital or even in many university centers.

A prime example is the new trend in coronary artery bypass operations. These are the operations that divert blood around a blocked region of a heart artery in an attempt to return the blood supply to the heart. The operation seems to reduce the pain (angina) associated with coronary artery disease. Despite earlier hopes, current data suggest that the operation may not prolong life in those who suffer from coronary artery disease. There is little question, however, that it does improve the quality of life. Patients who were in almost constant distress can become pain free. Where the operation is performed has little effect on the long-term survival of the patient—even the five-year results at the "best" centers are discouraging. However, where the operation is performed and who does it has two profound short-term effects: the less able centers have both far higher early mortality rates and less success in controlling anginal pain.

From a nucleus of several active centers, including the Cleveland Clinic, the Texas Heart Institute, and Baylor University, the procedure has spread like wildfire to every major hospital in the country. Hospitals and surgeons have jumped on the bandwagon, whether or not they are fully qualified or proficient enough to execute the procedures properly. The result is that the mortality rates, the complication rates, and the failures at some hospitals are far greater than those at the best places. In a sense this represents a public deception, for the unsuspecting, uninformed patient has no idea that his surgeon or his hospital may be poorly qualified to carry out the operation. How did this come about? Because there is no regulation at all over operative procedures. Anyone and any hospital can do them. What's more, there is tremendous pressure for a surgeon and a hospital to keep up with the latest trends. Patients want the procedures. Surgeons and hospitals want to make a living. They have a strong desire to forge ahead, even though their qualifications may be far below those of the hospital down the street. They probably are not intentionally offering marginal services. They do not consciously want to hurt patients. They may even rationalize that they are performing a necessary community service. But, whatever the motives, the results are the same. When a hospital or a surgeon performs a dangerous operation so infrequently that proficiency is never achieved, and does it despite the fact that a nearby facility is geared to do a superb job, both patients and the community are seriously wronged.

All level-three operations and diagnostic procedures are subject to these considerations. You may be referred to a surgeon and a hospital that does them, but do they do them well and often? Ask and investigate before you go ahead.

Certain hospitals are renowed for special expertise. We have already talked about the unique problems that children face. Children's hospitals can generally handle them best. There are special cancer hospitals like Sloan Kettering in New York, Roswell Park in Buffalo, M.D. Anderson in Houston. There are heart institutes and hospitals that enjoy outstanding reputations in cardiac surgery: the Texas Heart Institute in Houston, the Cleveland Clinic, and Stanford University Medical Center are a few. Some hospitals have special expertise in neurosurgery, complicated eye surgery, pediatric surgery, liver diseases, and rehabilitation. They can be found by conferring with your physician, with any friends who are doctors, or by looking through the medical journals to see where those who are writing about your particular problem and those who are editing the journals are located.

❦

NONTEACHING HOSPITALS

Hospitals in rural communities, small cities, or suburbs may not have medical students or postgraduate physician trainees. That does not make them bad places, but it does imply less sophistication and less specialization than one would expect to find at a teaching institution.

We have talked about the value of these hospitals for "routine" care. Many are excellent for everyday medical and surgical problems. When situations go beyond the routine and reach the second level, make very sure the hospital can take care of your special needs. If you ever have need of the intensive care or the coronary care unit, are doctors always available on the premises, specifically assigned to those patients—not to the emergency room? If you need the emergency facility, is the emergency room open round-the-clock and staffed full time by a qualified physician? If you have pediatric needs, how well can the hospital handle them? Do they have a pediatrician in the emergency room or on call? Do they have a separate pediatric floor with trained pediatric nurses? If you cannot get satisfactory answers to these questions, and another better-staffed, better-equipped hospital is available, consider going there. If you live fifty miles from a more sophisticated medical center but your medical needs are pressing, you may have to settle for second best.

❦

OTHER METHODS OF EVALUATING HOSPITALS

We have discussed hospital size and teaching functions as measures of hospital sophistication. We have also discussed availability of special care facilities, physician manpower, the quality of emergency care. There are other criteria and other sources of information that can help you assess a hospital's quality.

Is it accredited? There is an organization known as the Joint

Commission on Accreditation of Hospitals (JCAH) which evaluates hospital performance and safety features and accredits the hospital or denies accreditation. Accreditation is no assurance of excellence, but it is one guideline. Lack of accreditation or recent loss of accreditation raises the question, Why? It may be that some of the hallways are in need of repair, that the records are not being kept up to date, that aging structures present some possible fire hazard. Or it may be that daily patient care is seriously deficient. There may not be enough physicians. The doctors at the hospital may be unlicensed. There may be an inadequate nursing staff. As of now patients are not privy to all of the findings of the JCAH, but by asking the hospital administration you can learn whether or not the hospital is accredited. If it is not, you will not be able to find out the reasons, but you will have grounds to consider another hospital.

The local rescue squad is another good source of information. If your community has a fire rescue squad with skilled paramedics, they are frequently well aware of hospital emergency services. We saw in an earlier story that the wife of a heart attack victim was advised by the paramedics to let them take her husband to the university hospital. They knew which was best equipped for his needs. Ask your rescue squad director about the local hospitals; particularly their emergency facilities and their critical care units.

Ask your doctor, your friends' doctors, and any other physicians or nurses you may know about the hospitals in your community. You can even call several physicians' offices. Tell them you are new in the area, and ask which hospital the doctor uses and why. You can ask the nurses and doctors you know best where they would go or where they would take their families if they needed to be in a hospital.

The local nursing association and organizations that supply nurses to hospitals may be able to offer some valuable information. They can help you with the following questions: Which hospitals have the best nurses? Are they RNs—registered nurses rather than practical nurses? Which hospitals have the highest nurse-to-patient ratio? Which have the lowest turnover of nurses? Which are staffed mainly by full-timers and which use many replacement nurses? High nurse-to-patient ratio and continuity of nursing care are both important in excellent patient management.

4

The Emergency Department: How to Cut Down on Your Frustrations

PLANNING AHEAD FOR EMERGENCIES

Knowing what to do, whom to call, and where to go in an emergency can be lifesaving. It isn't sufficient to say, "Well, I'll call my doctor," "I'll call an ambulance," "I'll just go to the hospital down the street." Some emergencies are too urgent to waste time calling your doctor. You can't call an ambulance quickly unless you have the appropriate number attached to your telephone. Some hospitals don't even have emergency rooms; or even if they do, they may close after 10:00 P.M.

Every family must preplan for emergencies. Preplanning begins with familiarizing yourselves with immediate first-aid measures that you can initiate while you await the arrival of an ambulance or before you head for the hospital. For example, your household should have a poison-control list strategically placed. These are available at many drugstores, and through most poison-control centers whose numbers you can find in the telephone directory. These lists describe all of the common household chemicals, and drugs. They tell you what to do if your child swallows any of them. First-aid techniques for other problems are available in courses sponsored by schools, hospitals, and fire rescue squads. Cardiopulmonary resuscitation (CPR) courses (to revive a heart attack victim) are becoming increasingly popular. Statistics show that they are responsible for saving the lives of many loved ones. Many books are available on first-aid techniques, and it is advisable to have one at home and to be familiar with its contents.

For people who live in remote areas, where a hospital may be forty minutes away, personal first-aid education is a true necessity. Unless you can actively intervene, valuable lifesaving time may may be lost when an emergency strikes. For those of you who live in metropolitan areas, an elementary understanding of first aid, particularly CPR, is valuable, but less essential. If help is only five minutes away, it is often wiser to summon it or to go there directly rather than to spend valuable minutes beginning home treatment.

The second step in preplanning is to know how to summon help or where to go for it. You should research ambulance services and emergency numbers. In many parts of the country 911 is now the universal emergency number. It connects you to an operator who asks you whether you need the police, the fire department, or an ambulance. You describe the problem, and the operator quickly dispatches an emergency vehicle for an urgent medical need. In many metropolitan areas the 911 call system has worked extremely well. The average time from call to ambulance arrival in the Washington, D.C., area, for example, is now five minutes. If your area does not have a 911 emergency call system, you must locate several alternative emergency transport services and keep their numbers by the telephone. These may include the local fire rescue squad or a private ambulance company. A few moments of preplanning—calling these sources, asking what services they provide, how long they take to arrive, what level of emergency training the attendants have—is worthwhile. After you have evaluated the services and selected the best ones, you must keep their numbers readily available. In addition, your physician's office and home number should be handy. There may be times when your emergency may be serious but not life threatening, and you will want to call him first.

Finally, research the local hospitals. You should find out

which emergency rooms are best equipped and best staffed and the hours they are open.

Some hospitals may not even have an emergency room. Others may have one that operates only a few hours a day. Still others may have an emergency room with no physicians. When a patient comes in, a doctor may have to be called in from home. Others may have poorly qualified doctors or poor facilities to care for certain conditions. We saw in an earlier chapter that it is sometimes worth taking an extra five minutes to drive to a hospital with a qualified doctor on the premises. This is why you owe it to yourself and your family to research the local emergency departments before an emergency arises. Note their hours. Are they staffed by physicians twenty-four hours a day? Are the doctors physically there? Who are the doctors? Do they have any training or professional experience beyond an internship? What sort of backup personnel are available? Are there qualified surgeons, anesthesiologists, cardiologists, pediatricians? In short, how well can the hospital handle any emergency needs?

Perhaps there is only one hospital in town. In that case, if certain facilities are lacking, you may work with the town government toward a change, but for now the one will have to do. Then all you need to know is if a doctor is always present. If not, in an emergency it pays to call your own doctor and to alert the emergency room that you are coming so that they can notify the physician-on-call. If there are a number of hospitals to choose from if may be worth it to take the additional few minutes to reach the best-equipped and best-staffed one.

∽❧∼

HOW TO DECIDE WHOM TO CALL

If your problem is serious but not life threatening, call your physician first. He will be able to decide whether he should see you in his office or in the emergency room, or perhaps he may refer you at once to the appropriate specialist. For example, assume little Jimmy fell out of a tree onto his outstretched wrist. The deformity shouts out the diagnosis loud and clear: he has a fracture. Your physician may want to give him a thorough checkup to rule out any other injury, and he may want a particular orthopedic surgeon who he feels is very competent to take care of the fracture. By calling your own doctor you can get a referral to the specialist from him, rather than from an unfamiliar physician in the emergency room. In addition, calling your doctor first may get you faster service. After the call your physician will likely have you go to the emergency room where either he or the on-duty physician will examine Jimmy. Once the X-rays are completed and the broken bone is seen on the film, the orthopedic surgeon will probably come in and take over. Or, if his office is nearby, he may ask you to bring your son there. All of this can be coordinated by your personal physician.

The main value of most emergency rooms is that they are open when physicians' offices are not; they are equipped with supplies of emergency equipment, such as X-ray machines, drugs, resuscitative devices; and they have access to the full range of hospital services, including consultant specialist physicians, labor and delivery rooms, and operating rooms. Your physician's office can't begin to offer this breadth of critical care supplies. In the case of true, serious emergencies, the hospital is far superior to your physician's office.

A life-threatening emergency leaves no time for phone calls to the doctor. If your husband collapses with a heart attack, your two-year-old swallows a bottle of aspirin, or your face is battered in an automobile accident, a call to your personal physician comes later. First it's a car or an ambulance ride to the nearest *adequately equipped, adequately staffed* emergency department. If you truly need emergency service, dial 911 (if you live in an area where this is the emergency number), or telephone an ambulance company or the rescue squad. If you have time, you, a friend, or a relative should notify the emergency department and tell them you're on your way. Most emergency vehicles have communication systems. They, too, stay in contact with the emergency room if they feel that urgent care is required. The nurse, having received their call, then announces loudly, "Bad auto accident, three victims—gunshot wound of the chest—serious heart attack—severe head injury—

coming in." With that the emergency department team springs into action preparing to begin treatment the moment the ambulance arrives.

Another bit of advice: use ambulances wisely—only when you truly need them. Too often ambulances are used like taxicabs by patients without a pressing need. This makes them unavailable for those who are desperately in need, and if overdone, it causes the emergency department personnel to tune out the wall of the siren. There have been many instances when we have heard the sirens screech and seen the emergency room doors burst open dramatically. There on the stretcher lay a man with a stubbed toe, a child with a minor cat scratch, or a teen-ager with sunburn.

UNDERSTANDING THE EMERGENCY DEPARTMENT

The emergency department is the most frightening and intimidating section of large city hospitals. The screaming of sirens, the scurrying of personnel from place to place, the cries of patients in pain, the distress of relatives at the news of a death convey an aura of drama and urgency. In this atmosphere of perpetual crisis you may feel cowed and unnaturally submissive. If you are like most patients, you are torn by conflicting emotions: you may sit back timidly waiting your turn, trying to stay out of the way; you may feel relief knowing that you will soon get the care you need. At the same time your annoyance and even hostility may mount at the apparent lack of concern of the emergency room staff and the interminable wait that you are forced to endure. It is this strange dichotomy of the emergency department—lifesaving heroics on the one hand, seeming coldness and insensitivity on the other—that confuses most patients and provokes resentment. There is no part of the hospital that generates more complaints from patients.

⚜

THE UNIQUE PSYCHOLOGY OF EMERGENCY DEPARTMENT PERSONNEL

Perhaps it shouldn't be so, but the fact is that nurses and doctors who spend all of their working hours in the emergency room become somewhat anesthetized to suffering. This is particularly true in very busy emergency departments where the constant flow of people and the repetitive, mechanical responses to patients' problems have a dehumanizing effect. The desk clerk, the nurse, the physician begin to view patients as walking conditions that need repair, rather than as suffering human beings. If you understand this basic premise and appreciate the psychology of emergency department personnel, you will be able to function more effectively and obtain the best care possible in this setting.

Emergency medicine, unlike any other form of medical practice, demands immediate, automatic reactions, with robotlike precision. The physician and nurse must concentrate on starting the intravenous lines, resuscitating failing hearts, stopping life-threatening bleeding, providing oxygen to patients who can't breathe themselves, and setting up increasingly complex monitoring equipment. To do this efficiently and flawlessly, they must blank out the wails and moans of patients and family. If they don't, if they personally feel pain when they insert needles or introduce uncomfortable tubes into their patients' bodies, they can become inhibited and ineffectual in their lifesaving duties. Thus the efficient handling of life and death emergencies, of necessity, builds an emotional barrier between medical pracitioners and their patients.

Other aspects of emergency room life take their toll on the sensitivities of those who work there. Life-and-death emergencies are brief punctuations in the hours of dull repetition. For you, the patient, this may be the first broken bone you've ever had. The clerk, the nurses, the aids, the doctors have seen fifteen that day, one hundred that week, five thousand that year. You find it an anguishing, painful experience. For them it's another humdrum routine fracture. They can no longer feel your pain.

Finally, in busy emergency departments, the personnel work very hard. At the end of a shift their energy is drained, their nerves are jangled, and most remnants of compassion have faded away. I vividly recall my experiences as an intern at the Johns Hopkins Hospital in Baltimore. I would recoil in horror at the masses of people that packed the emergency department. When I entered my internship I listened intently to patient's cries for help, but several fifteen-hour days took their toll. Though I resisted, I found myself beginning to care mostly about the mechanics: suturing the lacerations, diagnosing appendicitis, putting in tubes, pumping hearts that had stopped beating by themselves. Patients' fears, concerns, pain, suffering, and annoyances became secondary to the things that had to be done.

To a great extent, emergency medicine blunts the sensitivities of the health-care providers and builds an emotional barrier between the physician and his patient. The kind of doctor-patient rapport that you hopefully have and can expert from your family physician generally won't be found in an emergency department. There are a few exceptions. The quiet small-town emergency room may be more like your doctor's office. There the unrushed staff, rarely assaulted by major disasters, may come through with their empathy intact. Even amid the frantic activities of a busy hospital emergency room an exceptional nurse or physician may have salvaged a good portion of his compassion.

This seemingly callous discussion may strike a raw nerve. "Just another doctor making excuses for his unfeeling colleagues," you think. Remember, our intention is to make you an informed consumer and an active participant in your health care. Understanding the inner workings and deep-rooted psychology of a very important section of the hospital—the area with which you will probably have the greatest contact—is a vital part of your hospital education. This does not mean that you have to accept rude treatment. You have a right to expect and demand that you be treated courteously and that your dignity be respected. There is no excuse for nastiness. If any of the emergency department staff treats you discourteously, make your feelings known. A gentle chide, such as "I realize that you are busy, but I have a problem too, and I would appreciate being treated courteously," will, if nothing else, remind the nurse, clerk, doctor, or whoever was rude, that his or her behavior was distasteful. If you are subjected to extreme rudeness, you may want to report this to the hospital administration. Be sure to note the name of the offender. Later write, call, or have a personal interview with the hospital administrator to describe and discuss the incident.

Another problem that you may face is the frank disregard for privacy and dignity that occurs too often in the emergency department. Unless they are reminded, the nurses and doctors, out of habit, convenience, or simply from thoughtlessness, may put their patients on public display. They may leave curtains open or partially drawn with patients unclad or not fully clad. This violation of your self-respect can be very distressing. You don't have to put up with it. Insist that you be covered when you are not being examined and that your door be closed or your curtains drawn.

HOW TO ASSESS THE KIND OF EMERGENCY ATTENTION YOUR PROBLEM DESERVES

In order of priorities, emergency departments are geared to (1) spring rapidly and efficiently into action to save lives immediately endangered; (2) uncover and head off illnesses or injuries that might become life threatening; (3) manage emergency problems that are not dangerous but that require some treatment and relief from suffering; (4) evaluate and treat minor everyday ailments; (5) see patients with chronic, long-standing complaints. As you progress down the list, you move lower down on the scale of relative urgency. Your wait will probably reflect this. As you enter categories 4 and 5, you get out of the realm of true emergencies and shift into a new sphere: problems that most emergency departments are not interested in and categorize as "nuisance" visits. These non-emergency problems, such as minor colds and two-year-old back-aches, often evoke a response that is more than dispassionate—it may be downright rude. As indicated earlier you should not be treated this way, and if you are, you have the right to make your dissatisfaction known—to the head nurse, the doctor, or later (via a letter or personal visit) to the hospital administrator.

The following is a valuable piece of advice that will help you, and your community, and will enable the emergency department to do the best job possible with minimal unpleasantness for all: Don't use the emergency department as a replacement for your private doctor. Problems that are long-standing or that can wait for a visit to your doctor's office should be cared for there.

If you're in shock as the result of a car accident, if your husband or wife is ashen and unconscious from a heart attack, if your child's asthma makes her gasp for air, you will generally get help the moment you enter the emergency room door, assuming, of course, there is a physician on duty. The nurse or physician out front will recognize a life-threatening need and will expedite your care. In addition, those who arrive by ambulance are seen, at least briefly, the moment they reach the emergency room.

The only illnesses or injuries which command this kind of instant action are those where seconds count, not to spare you discomfort but to save your life. Profuse bleeding, profound internal injuries, severe heart attacks, rapidly falling blood pressure (shock), deep coma, and blockage of the air passages (which can cause asphyxiation) are a few examples of situations that demand instant attention.

The second order of emergency room problems encompasses those that are potentially serious but are not yet urgent. The child with severe pain in her abdomen may have appendicitis. Time counts; too long a delay, can mean rupture, peritonitis, and transformation of a relatively minor problem into a very grave one. Here it isn't seconds but minutes and hours that spell the difference between a successful and tragic outcome. The child needs to be seen shortly after she arrives. She can then wait for the appropriate X-rays, blood tests, and specialist consultation. In fact, some wait and observation may be helpful in the evaluation. Physicians can tell a great deal by observing changes over a period of time. What was at first an uncertain diagnosis may become clear-cut in an hour or two.

The same is true for the individual who has injured his head in a fall or his abdomen in a moderately severe auto crash. As long as he is alert, not in shock, and not in immediate danger, instant attention isn't mandatory; but prompt attention and close observation are. Otherwise the physicians may be caught off guard when suddenly confronted with shock from a hemorrhaging liver or deep coma from the pressure of bleeding inside the skull.

Third in our order of emergency room priorities are illnesses and injuries that demand treatment, may be utterly miserable or excruciatingly painful but have little or no chance of causing a fatal collapse at once or ever.

These conditions, which cause moaning, wailing, vomiting, and writhing, will be taken care of. How rapidly can depend on whether your private physician meets you in the emergency room or how busy the emergency room physician is. It is these conditions that cause the greatest friction between patients and health care providers.

Nowhere in the practice of medicine is the chasm between patient expectations and physician response wider. Here the physician's objective, dispassionate approach to medical problems clashes with the personal needs and feelings of the patient. A child with a fractured bone is in pain, a woman with a stomach virus wretches uncontrollably, a young man with a four-inch stab wound across his arm begs for relief, the middle-aged man with a kidney stone moans in great distress. These people are hurting, are miserable, are in the emergency department because they want and need help. And they want it now! But to the staff they aren't first-order priority patients. If there are life-threatening cases that have to treated first, those patients, although uncomfortable, may have to wait. Understanding this, and even being thankful that your life isn't in danger, may temper your natural feelings of neglect, or even outrage, and make your wait easier to bear.

Patients in this third category often ask for medication while they wait to be seen and resent it when their wishes or demands are denied. There are two very important reasons why drugs cannot be given prior to a complete examination in an examining room. First, it isn't safe. Most medications produce drowsiness. A patient in a waiting area can fall off the chair and injure himself. Second, pain and other symptoms are important signals that complement the doctor's examination. It tells him where the problem is and gives vital clues about its severity. If pain and tenderness are obliterated by drugs, the doctor cannot carry out an accurate examination. A six-year-old boy was once brought to me who had suffered severe abdominal pain earlier that evening. His mother gave him some codeine—a strong pain reliever—that she had around the house. When I saw the child he was resting comfortably and was barely tender in his lower abdomen. I was concerned enough to admit him to the hospital and order a battery of laboratory tests. Finally, after six hours, when the effects of the codeine wore off, the hallmark signs of appendicitis showed up. We quickly operated, just before the appendix ruptured. His mother, out of the loving desire to comfort her ailing son, had masked the diagnosis and nearly caused a major injury.

The case above was a valid emergency, but today emergency room visits involve so many nonurgent problems that some very busy city hospitals have provisions or separate facilities to care for them. They may divide patients, at the door, into urgent and nonurgent care and direct them either to the regular emergency room or to a routine care minor clinic. Smaller hospitals, however, can't support separate facilities. All patients who come to their emergency rooms are cared for by the same team of nurses and physicians. Patients with minor colds or three-month-old knee pains are seen after all those in urgent need or in serious acute pain are taken care of.

∾❦∾

WHAT TO DEMAND AND HOW TO EXPEDITE EMERGENCY CARE

What you can expect and must demand from a emergency department is efficient, thorough, competent management of your illness or injury. If the situation is urgent or life threatening, you have the right to immediate attention. If it is not, you can expect no more than to be taken in turn after those in more serious straits are attended to. First, you must accurately assess your needs. Second, if your wait is excessive, you have several alternatives.

Try to see yourself as others (in this case, the emergency room personnel) see you. It isn't easy. You hurt; you are miserable; you want relief. They are busy; they've seen thirty people that day with precisely what you've got; and they are frantically trying to save four dying patients. How urgent is your need?

If your child is turning blue in the waiting area or your husband, who was plunked in a back corner, has just crumpled to the floor clutching his chest, there is no question that you call for help. Inform the receptionist and nurse as quickly as possible. Your problem is now a bona fide life-and-death emergency that requires urgent care.

Perhaps you or a relative is suffering greatly from a non-life-threatening injury or illness. The place may be packed with wall-to-wall people. You can be sure that you've got a long wait. Without question you have the right to ask the nurse or receptionist approximately how long a wait you might expect. Speaking courteously, without being accusatory, will probably be effective in getting a straight answer. If the wait is more than you can endure, you have several choices. The best alternative is to call your family physician. He might be able to meet you there or summon the required specialist—for example, an orthopedist for a probable fracture. This will save you time. Remember, your doctor has more of a personal concern for your needs, either life threatening or "just" physically distressing, than does the emergency room staff. Another option is to call a nearby hospital. See if there is a physician on duty and whether they are less backed up. A fifteen-minute trip to another facility may save you a three-hour wait.

HOW TO MAKE YOUR COMPLAINTS HEARD

What if you have no private doctor and there is nowhere else to go? What if you have accurately assessed your needs and expectations, looked around to appraise the ongoing activity in the emergency department, and reached the conclusion that you are being dealt with unfairly. What can you do?

Unlike a prolonged hospital stay where you have daily access to the hierarchy of command—the nursing supervisor, the patient grievance representative, the hospital adminstrator—a one-time visit to an emergency department, when your needs are pressing, leaves less time to act and fewer courts of appeals. If you yell and scream, rant and rave, you will either be ignored, intentionally moved down the patient list, or if you are grossly disruptive or obstreperous, physically removed by the hospital security team or the police (I have seen this happen on several occasions). It is definitely to your advantage to keep your cool.

If your wait seems excessive for no apparent reason, ask to see the head nurse. Don't confront the desk clerk. She has nothing to do with the medical care. Ask the nurse what the problem is. Is it too few physicians, too many patients, not enough beds, very sick patients that are hidden from your view and are taking a lot of time, unavailability of the physician or appropriate technicians, or an oversight—that they have simply forgotten you? Posing reasonable questions and paying close attention to answers should put this situation into perspective. You may find out why you're waiting, whether or not the answer is accurate. At least you should learn approximately how much longer you may have to wait. You will also have announced your presence and your concerns to the nurse, who now knows you are there. Each time you confront her she'll be more acutely aware of the duration of your wait.

Keep in mind that, for the most part, if you are forced to wait a long time, there is some reasonable explanation. Contrary to what patients may sometimes believe, the hospital and its staff have no personal vendettas against you and no nefarious reasons to make you unhappy. In fact, they are as anxious to clear everybody out as you are to be taken care of. The majority of long waits are simply traffic jams. The facilities and personnel can't handle everyone fast enough to keep patients happy. Alternatively, of course, they may simply be inefficient or unduly slow. At the moment you are sitting there, there isn't much you can do about this except those things we have suggested: diplomatically making your presence felt; calling your own doctor; or going to another emergency department. Later, however, you and other disgruntled friends in the community should cry out for a change. Discuss the problem with the emergency department director, the hospital administrator, the chairman of the hospital board. Public pressure is an important determinant of hospital policy because hospitals are economically dependent on community support. If the right people are made aware of problems in the emergency department, they'll make changes. Perhaps expansion of the physical plant, the addition of more nurses or doctors, or more expeditious laboratory or X-ray examinations are the solution. Making your voice heard and encouraging others to do the same will stimulate the hospital to make appropriate improvements, so that your next visit is less distressing.

Once you've been "taken" into the treatment room, there may be other waits that are unavoidable and, at times, even necessary. These take place once you're through your initial examination. After the doctor sees you, he may order X-rays, laboratory tests, special consultations with other physicians. Each of these processes takes time as you can surely see. If it's late at night, technicians may have to be called in from home. During the day there are others in line for X-rays and often stacks of blood and urine waiting in the laboratory for testing. The consultation specialist may be finishing his appointments in his office forty minutes away. All of these special needs may, therefore, take time.

As we mentioned before, time is sometimes a valuable adjunct in diagnosis. The way that physical findings change or the way you respond to some initial therapy can tell the physician a great deal about problems. Examining you three times in a three-hour period rather than only once may make the difference between discharging you prematurely or uncovering a serious illness. So for some conditions, waiting, however unpleasant, may be lifesaving. Waits for test results can be less tedious if a friend or a relative can join you. Visitors may not be permitted during the initial examination, but companions may be welcome during the waiting phase. Which brings us to another pet peeve of many emergency department users—policies regarding friends and relatives.

ॐ

WHAT ROLES VISITORS CAN PLAY IN EMERGENCY CARE

Almost nobody likes to give up his sick friend or relative when his name is called. Parents don't want to leave children. Middle-aged people don't want to abandon their elderly parents. A young man doesn't want to entrust his girl friend to these strangers and this unfeeling place. However, for the sake of harmony, to avoid utter chaos, and for other, equally compelling reasons, it isn't possible or advisable for every patient to bring a companion into the examining area.

Here again it is important to assess your needs and desires and to be reasonable. Generally, except in the case of parents with small children, the nurse or physician won't want nonpatients in the examining room. The reasons range from pure habit and utter capriciousness to very good ones: a friend or relative standing by may actually inhibit or embarrass the patient, thereby complicating the history-taking or examination; if emergency, lifesaving therapy is required, extra people, particularly ones who are emotionally involved, can get in the way both physically and psychologically; most emergency departments aren't sufficiently large to handle crowds—one or two visitors with each patient doubles or triples the volume of people and is disruptive; finally, in most emergency departments there is very little privacy—flimsy curtains often separate rows of patients, and it can be embarrassing and degrading for other patients to stretch out before a parade of strangers. In short, unless there is a pressing need, visitors should generally remain in the waiting area while the patient is being examined.

There are, however, valid times and reasons for a friend or a family member to come along. When these reasons exist, you shouldn't let blanket, inflexible hospital rules immobilize you. For example, you may be accompanying a retarded child or adult, a senile parent, a deaf or mute friend who can't communicate his problems. Your mouth and ears may be an important link between him and the physician. You may be with your arthritic, slightly senile mother who, if left unattended, will surely climb out of bed, fall, and get hurt. She may need your constant supervision. Perhaps you are with a friend who, after taking an overdose of sleeping pills, is deeply comatose. Historical details, including the nature and amount of pills taken, the time that they were swallowed, and your friend's past problems, are vital information. Your communicating with the doctor is essential. After you have told him what you know, however, there may be no valid reason for you to stay with your friend while the treatment is under way.

As with waiting times, let reason and understanding be your

guide here. If you feel that you have a good reason to accompany your friend or relative, inform the nurse. If she refuses to let you in, find our why. Are her reasons better than yours? If not, ask to speak with the doctor and discuss the matter with him or her. In most cases, if your friend or relative truly needs you, you will be allowed in. If you reach an impasse, you have several choices: call the emergency room director or hospital administrator if it is during working hours; call your own physician; go to another hospital, or simply walk in uninvited. The problem with the latter is that it may backfire. You may generate such hostility that your friend or relative is ignored. Only in the most extreme cases, if you strongly believe your loved one is in jeopardy without you, should you barge in against instructions. If the need isn't that compelling, swallow your pride and take up your grievance later with the hospital authorities. If there are flaws in their emergency department policies, they'll be anxious to work toward future solutions.

⁕

CHILDREN'S EMERGENCIES

Recently we saw a case involving a two-year-old child who had swallowed a bottle of his mother's mood elevating pills. Serious poisoning was inevitable in view of the amount taken and the diminutive size of the child. Not realizing that this was not the best choice, the parents whisked the child off to the doctor's office. The pediatrician began certain emergency procedures, but in moments the child developed seizures and had a cardiac arrest. He could not be saved. We are not certain that he would have been saved had the parents taken him to the hospital instead, but we do know that the chances would have been far greater. There, emergency equipment would have been available. He could have been placed on a respirator, given lifesaving drugs, and, perhaps, revived. The physician did not have those resources on hand; nor do most physicians.

Children's problems are particularly treacherous. As we noted in Chapter 2, children have special needs and require specialized evaluation. Even if your local hospital is competent to deal with most adult emergencies, it may not be equipped to handle children. The physician may be a surgeon or an internist and may simply be unfamiliar with pediatric emergencies. The rooms may not have child-sized tubes or other appropriate devices. The X-ray department may be poor at taking children's X-rays. The child stands the best chance of excellent care in a children's emergency room. As Samuel J. Tibbits, board chairman of the American Hospital Association, points out, "Wise parents should check the hospitals in their communities right now to find one with a pediatric emergency room. If you can't locate one, try to find a hospital emergency room near you that has a pediatrician on call. There is no substitute for pediatric skill when your child's life is at stake." Again, the urgency of the situation or the nature of your community may force you to take your child to the nearest facility. But if you have any choice at all, look for an emergency room that is well prepared to handle pediatric catastrophes.

WHAT TO DO IF YOU ARE DISSATISFIED WITH THE TREATMENT

What if you are dissatisfied with your emergency room evaluation? You bring in your two-year-old daughter, complain to the doctor that she has had a fever of 104 degrees for four days, is listless, isn't eating anything, and appears terribly sick to you. The doctor gives her a momentary glance, touches her back with his stethoscope, and says, "She just has a mild viral infection. Give her fluids and aspirin and call your own doctor tomorrow."

Your instincts tell you that his examination was cursory, that some lab tests were probably in order, and that he simply was not as thorough as you think he should have been. Unfortunately this sequence of events is not too uncommon. In fairness, there are two possible explanations. The doctor may be very good at recognizing childhood illnesses and also far more objective than you. He may be absolutely right. Your dissatisfaction may be because this is *your* child, and you are inexperienced with children's diseases. On the other hand, you may be right. Perhaps the doctor was too cavalier, too superficial, and too unconcerned. Whichever of you is correct, follow your instincts. Assume, if you believe it to be so, that the examination was inadequate. One can never be too safe. A few blood tests, a chest X-ray, a careful examination—even a spinal tap (if done by someone with experience)—are safe procedures. Unless you feel comfortable with the extent of the examination and the adequacy of testing, don't stop there. First, explain your concerns to the doctor. Let him know that you believe your child is quite sick and needs a careful evaluation. If he won't do any more, ask him if he is a pediatrician or, if not, whether he can call one. If he won't call your own and explain the situation to him, or take your child to the nearest pediatric hospital if you have access to one.

The same might be true for an adult examination. What if you drive your fifty-year-old husband, who has a history of heart disease, to the neighborhood emergency room. You tell the physician that he experienced severe chest pain that lasted one hour and was sweating and felt faint. By now the pain has largely dissipated. The physician takes a brief look and declares, "Looks like he's OK now. Take him home."

You believe, and rightly so, that he should have an electrocardiogram. The doctor, convinced that there is no clinical evidence of a heart attack, refuses. You are dissatisfied. Your immediate options are to call your own doctor or to take him elsewhere. You should do one of those things, for your instincts are correct. He should have an electrocardiogram. Later you or your doctor should contact the hospital administrator to appraise him of the shortcomings in that emergency room.

We don't mean to imply that the patient knows more than the doctor or that you should never trust the physician's decisions or recommendations. If patients could handle their own medical problems, they wouldn't need us at all. What we are saying is that you have a certain degree of innate intelligence and common sense. The fact that you are placed in an unfamiliar or awesome medical environment, manned by someone with a stethoscope and white coat, shouldn't subvert your reason. If something is grossly improper, you can sense it. If a doctor is unattentive, hurried, careless, overlooking important facts, you can tell. If you believe that certain well-known simple tests should be performed—an electrocardiogram, a urine test, a blood count, a chest X-ray—at least the doctor should be able to explain, to your satisfaction, why he didn't order those. Finally, if you are dissatisfied, you surely have the right to a second opinion and an examination by someone else. The findings may be precisely the same, but you will have reassured yourself and your family.

❧

MISUSING THE EMERGENCY ROOM

You shouldn't take all of your health problems to the emergency room. In recent years, hospital emergency rooms have become the primary care facilities for everyday illnesses. The majority of patients seen in most emergency facilities have colds, sore throats, aches and pains, chronic complaints of weakness and dizziness, burning on urination, vaginal discharges, longstanding swelling in their extremities, and mild fevers. They use the emergency room instead of the private physician. This presents several problems. First, all of these conditions can be checked out in the doctor's office in a regular scheduled visit. You can always ask for an urgent examination if the need is pressing. Second, these conditions will probably require ongoing management that only the private physician can provide. The emergency room is continually changing physicians. Bringing these problems time after time to the emergency setting leaves you without an ongoing manager; continuity with a single physician is an important part of good care. Third, crowding the emergency room with non-emergency problems denies others access to emergency care in times of true need. If the emergency physician is busy treating four colds and three long-standing strained backs, he can't respond promptly to someone with a heart attack. If you were that someone, you wouldn't want your life to be jeopardized by others who placed improper demands on the emergency room personnel and facilities. Finally, emergency room visits are quite expensive—much more than a visit to your doctor's office. Unless the condition is truly an emergency, most insurance policies, including Blue Shield and others, won't pay the hospital bill. On the other hand, some will pay for a visit to the doctor's office.

5

Hospitals Away From Home

A few years ago my sister was traveling cross-country with a group of friends. They were all about nineteen and in college. Everything was going smoothly until they hit Kansas; not that there is anything wrong with Kansas, but it happened to be there where my sister got something in her eye. So what? What's the big deal about something in an eye? For a contact-lens wearer, as my sister is, a cinder in the eye can get under the lens and scratch the cornea: a terribly painful ordeal and if not treated promptly and properly, a potentially dangerous state of affairs.

By the time she and her friends pulled into the nearest emergency room, her eye was massively swollen, bright red, and excruciatingly painful. It was a tiny hospital located somewhere in Kansas farm country. The moment my sister and her friends entered the hospital door the welcome mat was rolled up and stuffed into a corner. Everyone there, from the clerk at the desk, to the emergency room nurse, to the doctor who ultimately saw her, made it crystal clear that she and her "motley coed group" didn't belong there. My sister's college friends weren't disruptive, loud, rude, or in any way demanding or unpleasant. Even given the fact that they looked different, being long-haired, eastern, of mixed gender, and grimy from their week of camping, there was no cause to treat them with utter disgust and disdain.

My sister's traveling companions, who provided her only solace during this painful experience, were summarily dismissed from the waiting room. They were literally thrown out. My sister was abruptly ushered into an examining room where a middle-aged general practitioner, after whispering some very audible epithets to the nurse, approached her. The first three or four minutes of his ministrations to this patient-in-need consisted of lecturing her, chiding her, and making various inappropriate comments about "hippies and no-good kids today." Finally he got to her eye. With all the finesse of a gorilla, he poked, pulled, and in the crudest, most painful manner possible, attempted to pry open her swollen lid. She shrieked with pain but each shriek seemed to increase his fervor. It was almost as if he were enjoying hurting her. Finally, no closer to examining her eye or to removing her contact lens than when he started, he gave up and decided to admit her to the hospital.

That night, in this institution supposedly devoted to the needs of suffering people, was the most harrowing of my sister's life. After complaining for hours she was finally given some pain medication by a reluctant and equally prejudiced nurse. The nurse forced some drops in her eyes and my sister was finally able to remove her own contact lens. It soon became clear that not only was she unwelcome there but they had no resources to care for her properly. Or, perhaps, they refused to make them available. Either there were no ophthalmologists (eye physicians) in town or the physician who admitted her simply didn't call one. We never did learn which was true.

The solution to my sister's health problem, managed so ineptly and with such malice in this hostile town hospital, came later that night. She called my father, a professor at an eastern medical school, who had many medical colleagues. He called the chairman of the ophthalmology department at his school who spoke to the physician in the Kansas hospital. He then made arrangements with a colleague of his at the nearest major university medical center to see her the next day. It wasn't close—Denver, Colorado, to be exact—but the trip was essential.

The next day my sister departed from this unfriendly hospital and set out with her friends for Denver. She was seen at once by a professor of ophthalmology who treated her corneal abrasion, saw her on several occasions for the next few days, and then bid her farewell. Her eye healed, but the trauma of that hospital experience in Kansas will remain forever.

Hopefully, if you find yourself in a hospital far away from home, you won't suffer these indignities. Treatment like this is anathema to the sacred trust that hospitals, nurses, and physicians owe to the public. But even if your treatment is more compassionate, you may find that the hospital where you end up doesn't have the personnel or the resources to handle your needs. What can you do?

cℰ🙰

FINDING THE BEST HOSPITAL IN AN AWAY-FROM-HOME EMERGENCY

If you are lucky enough, as my sister was, to have a relative who is a physician or who works at a medical school, you can call him or her for advice. If not, you can call your own physician at home. Ask your doctor for a referral. He may know someone personally in that area. If he doesn't, at least he'll know which medical center in the vicinity is a quality place. Assuming you can travel, you can go directly there, or call the department that you need and ask that one of the physicians anticipate your arrival. They may not be willing or able to assign a specific physician on the basis of your phone call, but they will be able to tell you where to go when you arrive and how best to expedite your transfer.

If you don't have a personal physician or a friend who is a physician, or you are unable to contact your doctor, you can head for the nearest local city and find the largest hospital, preferably a university hospital, if the city has one.

You may be so seriously ill or injured or incapacitated that immediate transfer is out of the question. You may need urgent surgery or treatment and cannot be moved. You, if you can communicate, or your traveling companion should make every effort to get the best attention while you are there. Ask for a referral to the relevant board-certified or, at least, board-eligible physician. That may be a general surgeon, an orthopedic surgeon, neurosurgeon, internist, pediatrician, etc. If the right specialist is unavailable, ask for the physician who is most qualified at that hospital to care for you.

Arranging a Transfer

Once the acute crisis has passed, your next decision is when and if to request a transfer. You may feel comfortable where you are, pleased with your progress, and may want to stay. On the other hand, you may have a complication or a problem that is difficult to treat and that cries out for more sophisticated facilities. Or you may simply want to spend your convalescent period in a hospital closer to home. In general, physicians in a small-town hospital do appreciate the limitations of their medical environments. They are generally willing, even anxious, to send you where you will have access to specialists and a full range of medical services. The doctor who is caring for you there might suggest a referral to the nearest university hospital. He can, if you and he concur, arrange for admission there, to the service of the proper specialist, and an ambulance transfer. You and your doctor may disagree. He may want you to stay; you may want to go. It helps to bring a friend or relative and his or your local physician into the decision-making process. You're in no condition to think clearly or to negotiate. Others, not incapacitated, and particularly professional advisers, are invaluable. A full delineation of your problem, your doctor's reasons for wanting you to stay, and the pros and cons of transfer should lead to a meeting of minds. At the end you may both agree amicably to send you elsewhere; or you may agree to stay, recognizing that the doctor's reasons are compelling. You may, on rare occasion, vehemently disagree with your doctor's adamant position and decide to leave against his advice. If it comes to that, and hopefully it won't, you take a chance; for if you leave contrary to his advice, you are on your own. You, not the physician, become legally responsible if anything goes awry during the transfer process. If he can prove that he objected to your move, the doctor absolves himself of any liability should a mishap occur on route. Moreover, it may be impossible to get an ambulance service for an unauthorized transfer.

The ease with which you can get to a hospital nearer to home obviously depends upon two things: how sick you are and how far away you are. Regarding your physical ability to travel, the same considerations mentioned above apply here. As far as distance is concerned, a trip may or may not be practical.

A fifty- or seventy-five-mile ambulance ride is possible for those who are sufficiently stable to make the trip. Distances much beyond that may require air transfer. This process is no problem to arrange if you are in good condition. Your family member or the nurses simply make airline reservations and then transfer arrangements for the trip to and from the airport. The airline may want to confer with your physician to be certain that you aren't in any jeopardy or in need of special care. This transfer process is practical for individuals who are completely stable but who need long-term convalescent care—for example; a stroke victim. A family member can accompany such a person on the ambulance ride to the airport, the wheelchair transfer to the plane, and the ambulance trip to the destination hospital.

For patients who are in worse physical condition, air transfer can sometimes be arranged, but the process is more tedious. We have arranged air transfer for patients who were semiconscious and had intravenous fluids. Doing that takes a well-coordinated effort by physician and family member. The airline will accept a patient like that if an official, after talking to the physician, is confident that the patient is in no imminent danger, that the stewardesses will not have any major nursing functions to carry out, and that the patient can sit up or recline in an airline seat. The patient will generally be transported in the first-class section where there is more room, often at no additional (above the tourist) charge to the family.

We have been involved in the air transport of even sicker patients who, although not imminently in danger, had the potential of needing medical attention in flight. In some cases the family can arrange such a transfer if a doctor or nurse accompanies the patient. Obviously, this creates logistical problems and can be quite costly, but the persistent and insistent family can work with the airlines and the hospital to make these arrangements. Unfortunately these transportation arrangements aren't part of everyday hospital life. The hospital may or may not be familiar with the mechanisms involved. Often the major coordinating responsibilities are left to the family's devices. If you are faced with this difficult and unusual problem, begin your transfer arrangements via the attending physician. Ask him what in-flight equipment will be needed and who should be at the side of the sick traveler. Then you will have to provide the nurse or physician traveling companion. The hospital administrator can assist here. Finally, once the medical details are ironed out, you and the physician will have to find an air carrier that will accept the patient. This may even require hiring the services of a private airline company rather than utilizing a standard commercial carrier.

PREPLANNING FOR TRAVEL AWAY FROM HOME

No one likes to consider the possibility of illness or an injury during a vacation or business trip, but they may occur. When you travel be sure to carry identification, and by all means, have some insurance information handy in your wallet. Generally, most medical insurance companies provide a card that gives basic insurance information, including your policy number and expiration date. Don't leave home without a current card strategically placed where you or the hospital personnel (should you be incapacitated) can find it. Also carry with you the name or names and numbers of people to contact in the event of an emergency and the name and number of your hometown doctor.

If you are elderly of if you have a particular health problem, more preplanning may be in order. Some health data—from a simple Med Alert card describing your condition (epilepsy, heart disease, diabetes) to more extensive information, including actual hospital summaries, records from your physician, recent electrocardiogram tracings, and a full list of all medications you are taking— offer valuable guidance for any new physician who may have to care for you. It's worth the effort to gather this information and carry it with you when you travel. If you suffer serious health problems, you may even want to research the local health care facilities before you go. Additional guidance can come from your local physician. He may have valuable suggestions concerning the best hospitals in the areas where you'll be traveling. He may even be able to give you the names of good physicians he knows personally or by reputation in those locales.

❧

WHAT TO DO IF YOU GET SICK IN A HOTEL

Most large hotels, particularly the large chains, have doctors on call. For routine health care needs they will come to your room and perform usual house-call services. If your problem is more urgent, the hotel operator will usually have ready access to emergency transport numbers. Call her and tell her that you urgently need an ambulance.

❧

WHAT TO DO IF YOU GET SICK WHILE TRAVELING ABROAD

Most of the larger European (both western and eastern) cities have relatively sophisticated medical care facilities. Many have hospitals known as "The American Hospital" that are staffed mostly by American physicians and that cater to American residents and travelers. In general, if they are available, they are your best bet. The quality of care is most uniform and the personnel speak English. Paris, France, Beirut, Lebanon, and many other large cities have these facilities. If there are no American Hospitals, you have two other prime options. First, you can contact the American consulate or Embassy and get a recommendation from them. Second, if there is an American military installation nearby, there may be a base hospital which will care for stricken American travelers.

6

Expediting Your Admission
to the Hospital

No matter how well prepared you are, entering a hospital can be disturbing. Your life-style and activites are disrupted and you are, naturally, apprehensive. This is also true for physicians about to be hospitalized, perhaps even more so. But it is important to keep in mind that such temporary disturbances are minor prices to pay for the potential reward of improved health and well-being.

The purpose of this chapter is to guide you through the admitting processes so that there will be a minimum of surprises awaiting you. It should prepare you for most of the initial hospital procedures, so that they will move more swiftly and smoothly for you.

There are two major types of hospital admissions: the emergency admission and the elective admission. Obviously an emergency admission would preclude many of the possible preparations: if you have been in an automobile accident, you're not going to have your toothbrush, pajamas, and favorite pillow immediately available.

Let us then discuss the elective admissions to the hospital. Later in the chapter we will give you additional pointers for emergency admissions.

e*

ELECTIVE ADMISSIONS

Mrs. J. P. White just left her physician's office. He told her that the X-rays of her gallbladder showed evidence of many small stones and that she will need a cholecystectomy (removal of the gallbladder). She advised her doctor that she had never had an operation before and therefore didn't know any surgeons. He recommended Dr. Jim Smith.

Dr. Smith's office scheduled operating time at County Memorial Hospital for June 2 at 8:00 A.M. They told Mrs. White that she would be admitted by 2:00 P.M. on June 1 and that she needed several laboratory studies prior to admission. If she would stop by the office, they would give her a list of the necessary tests; or if she were brave enough to try to take down the medical terms, they could give her the list by phone. Generally this would be all of the information offered Mrs. White unless she asked additional questions.

What Routine Testing Is All About and How to Cut Down on Some of the Costs

The purpose of pre-admission testing (P.A.T.) is to establish a data base line within seventy-two hours of surgery and to avoid the unnecessary costs of an additional day of hospitalization prior to the operation. Your insurance policy will almost certainly cover this outpatient service.

Some of the routine laboratory and X-ray testing may be done once you have entered the hospital, but the trend in these days of cost containment is to do more and more in the outpatient setting. Every day spent in the hospital for tests that could just as well have been run beforehand adds an extra couple of hundred dollars to the cost. What's more, your insurance may not pay for those extra days: the financial burden may be yours alone. Today Blue Cross and the other third-party payers scrutinize all hospital bills. If they find extra hospital days simply for routine testing, they frequently won't pay. It behooves you, therefore, to know exactly what will and can be done before you are admitted and what must be done in the hospital. If you are going in for routine surgery, is your admission scheduled three days in advance to allow time for "routine" studies? If so, you'll want to consult your physician about the possibility of having those before you enter. Otherwise you'll have extra hospital days and, quite likely, a personal financial obligation.

If you are forty years of age, most hospitals require a complete blood count, which includes a white blood cell count; a red blood cell count, a microscopic description of your white blood cells; a hematocrit, a measure of the concentration of red cells in your blood (to tell whether or not you are anemic); and a urinalysis. Patients over forty or those with planned operations will often need the above base-line studies plus a chest X-ray, an electrocardiogram, and a complete chemical screen known as an SMA 12/60 or SMA 6/60. The blood tests tell us whether the various chemical components are normal or abnormal. These components include calcium, phosphorus, sodium, potassium, chloride, uric acid, cholesterol, various body enzymes, and other elements. These tests ensure that you are ready for an operation and that surgical and anesthesia risks are minimized. If you are not having an operation but are being evaluated for a specific medical problem, such as kidney, liver, lung, or heart problem, these studies help guide the physician toward a proper diagnosis, an effective treatment plan, and an assessment of your progress.

Some Basic Points About Accommodations

We will discuss the question of rooms and roommates in our Chapter 15 Hospital life. For now, let's just mention the admission routine.

Most insurance policies cover semiprivate rooms—usually two patients to a room. In most hospitals semiprivate rooms are now two-patient rooms, some are four, and a few still have as many as six, but this is most unusual in the "semiprivate" setting today. If you wish to have a private room, discuss this with your physician.

He may make the arrangements, or he may have you do this directly with the admitting office. Private rooms often have to be reserved some time in advance. Their limited supply rarely offers you a spur-of-the-moment vacancy. If you choose a private room, you will almost surely be responsible for the difference in cost, since insurance coverage is usually limited to semiprivate facilities. The hospital may insist that you pay that difference in advance. To avoid a surprise, check that point before you go. Ask the clerk at the admitting office.

Some hospitals not only give you a choice of semiprivate versus private, but also allow you to choose smoking or nonsmoking areas. You will probably not be able to choose your roommate, but if you have serious roommate problems, there are ways of switching rooms later. This, too, we will address in Chapter 15.

Information Needed by the Admitting Office and How to Supply It

This varies from hospital to hospital. Call the admitting office and ask what information will be needed and if you can phone it in. Most hospitals will want the following *five* items:

• The social security card or number of the head of the household (that person who will have the ultimate responsibility for the bill).

• Your insurance cards or numbers. (It is best to bring the cards with you. Many cards have several numbers that you probably won't know how to interpret, but the admitting officer will).

• Your Medicare and/or Medicaid card. (You may have private coverage as well as Medicare and/or Medicaid. It is important to bring all these insurance cards so that the total extent of your coverage will be clarified.)

• Name, address, and phone number of your employer and of your spouse. (The business office generally runs a verification of employment in order to guarantee any residual payments.)

• Name, address, and phone number of the person to notify in case of an emergency.

This is by no means an exhaustive list of the necessary admitting information, but they are the key items which may or may not be found in your wallet. By having this information readily available you will save a great deal of time and expedite the admission process.

What to Bring With You

The most frequently asked questions are whether the patient can bring a pillow, a TV set, or medications to the hospital. As a rule of thumb, if it doesn't fit into an overnight bag, don't bring it.

Take the items that you would need for routine comfort: toothbrush, toothpaste, deodorant, shaving equipment, pajamas or nightgown, robe, and slippers. Optional items might include makeup, hand or body lotion, stationery and stamps, address book, needlework projects, crossword puzzle books, perhaps a novel or two, and a TV guide.

Do not bring any electrical appliances! This includes your portable radio or TV, your bedside clock, the blow dryer, the plug-in electric razor. The hospital must adhere to very strict fire safety codes. Each electric outlet and plug is designed to reduce or eliminate any hazards to the patient. Generally there is no problem if your appliance is battery operated, but check with the admitting office to be safe and avoid embarrassment.

You may bring your own pillow or blanket, but there is a chance that it will end up in the hospital laundry or be misplaced. The hospital will not take responsibility for lost items, so mark your pillow boldly and, like Linus, carry your blanket with you. Seriously, many patients do not sleep well without their own pillow. We think it's worth the risk of loss in order to get adequate rest; just make sure it's clearly labeled!

Most hospitals will not allow patients to use their own medications. Safety and quality control demands that the hospital pharmacy and the nurses supply all drugs. If you do take medications regularly, bring a list. All of your doctors must know exactly what you have been taking. This will help them order drugs for you and will protect you from any potential dangerous drug interactions. If you do bring your medications from home, they will generally be returned to you before you leave. But occasionally they get lost, so it is best for you to bring in a written list. If you don't know the names and they aren't written on the bottles, bring the actual drugs along.

You will most likely continue taking many of your regular medications, such as vitamins, birth control pills, blood pressure medications, digitalis, insulin. Some of these and many others will be reevaluated and, perhaps, changed or modified in light of your current problem.

Bringing Work With You

When you are in the recovery phases and find that you have several comfortable hours a day, there is no earthly reason why you can't plan to do some simple office work. Don't expect to carry on extensive negotiations or stressful phone calls, and if you are in the hospital to get some real rest and to escape work pressures, office work may be best put aside. But otherwise some simple reading, writing, paper work can help pass monotonous hours, actually be therapeutic, and help speed your recovery and return to normal daily life.

One word of caution. Safeguard valuable papers when you are out of the room. One salesman planned to do some work after undergoing his brief hernia operation. His papers, organized on the bedside table, had disappeared when he returned. The housekeepers had neatly stacked them in a bottom drawer of his bedside table. The two unpleasant hours of anxiety that he went through before finding that his papers had not been thrown out were not conducive to rapid healing.

A Timesaving Tip

Bring a list of all previous hospitalizations, operations, major illnesses, allergies, and drug reactions. During the first hospital day either your doctor or the house staff doctor will be writing up your complete medical history. This takes a good deal of time and is usually quite thorough. If you have prepared this list of information carefully, head-scratching delays will be avoided.

The physician will also be asking questions about any previous family history of diabetes, cancer, tuberculosis, hereditary illnesses, and the age and cause of death of specific family members. Again, you can save time by having this information recorded on paper before your admission.

What to Do If You Are Planning an Elective Admission and You Have No Insurance

You will have to discuss your options beforehand with the business office. They can help you manage this big financial burden by initiating medical assistance (Medicaid) if you qualify, helping to arrange a bank loan, providing a charity care grant, or working out another payment mechanism. A private hospital may insist that uninsured patients pay a considerable amount in advance. This may seem callous and outside the humanitarian spirit of medical care. We won't get into a philosophical discussion of the pros and cons of this system. The fact, however, is that you may face two alternatives: come up with several hundred dollars at the time of admission or go to a publicly supported hospital. To avoid being turned away at the door, it is a good idea to investigate the hospital's policy and decide on a payment plan before you go.

Young couples about to have a family addition have nine months to investigate the financial arrangements. Many insurance policies don't cover obstetrics, or they may cover only a small portion. Here again the hospital may insist on some prepayment. Before the labor pains begin, you'd better examine your insurance policy and clarify the hospital's practice.

THE EMERGENCY ADMISSION

There is really no way to prepare for an emergency admission except to be sure that you always carry ample identification, including medical insurance information. Your spouse, family member, or close friend will have to provide the admitting office with all necessary information as soon as possible. The admitting office can wait; your treatment can't.

If you have no relative or informed friend to help, a hospital service representative will come to your room when you are able to communicate. He or she will obtain the pertinent information at that time.

Now that you've been admitted to the hospital, we'll try to familiarize you with the inner workings of this complex institution. The hospital is like a manufacturer; its produce is patient care, *your care*.

PATIENT CHECKLIST

1. Pre-admission testing—ask your doctor.

2. Room selection—call the admitting office, or discuss this first with your private physician. The hospital may want the request to come from him.

3. Admitting procedure—call the admitting office.
   a. Social security card or number of head of household.
   b. Insurance card or number.
   c. Medicare/Medicaid card.
   d. Name, address, and phone number of employer for self and spouse.
   e. Name, address, and phone number of person to notify in case of emergency.

4. List of allergies, medications you are taking, known drug reactions, previous hospitalizations, operations, major illnesses, and family history.

5. A list of items you are taking with you to the hospital. This is often required once you are admitted, and it is helpful when you check out.

6. Money—maximum ten dollars in cash.

7. Visitors and visiting hours—call the admitting office for details. (For a more detailed discussion, see Chapter 15.)

7

Understanding the Nursing Staff and How It Can Benefit You

It has often been said that good nursing care can be the single most important stimulus to prompt recovery. Nurses are taught not only the specific mechanical techniques necessary to their profession but also to be keen observers of any physical or psychological changes in their patients. Because of this training they are able to provide that extra measure of cheer and understanding that can add considerably to your general comfort. It should quickly be added, however, that not every nurse fits our idealized picture of an angel of mercy with unlimited time. Also, changes within the nursing profession are taking place more rapidly than in many other areas involving medical personnel, and the resulting changes in nursing duties may prove confusing to anyone not familiar with the modern scene. The very best way of assuring yourself good nursing care is, first of all, to understand who's who and who does what.

Fifty years ago the answer was simple. Hospitals had nurses and doctors. The doctors examined the patients, planned the treatment, and wrote orders. The nurse did everything else. She made the patient comfortable, gave him baths, brought and removed the bedpan, dispensed medications, fed him if necessary, took his temperature, and wrote notes for the doctor to see. There was no cast of characters. One nurse did all of these things.

Times have changed, and nurses have become more specialized. Today, except in very small hospitals, there is a hierarchy of nurses whose duties are as stratified as those of the employees of a large corporation.

There are nurses who are in charge. They rarely touch patients. There are nurses who dispense medications. There are nurses who do more menial things, such as make beds, give baths, and change bedpans. Finally, there are nurses who are superspecialized. They may be teachers. They may be managers of specific problems: after-discharge home care, psychiatric illnesses, intensive care, childbirth education, immediate postsurgical care, care of the newborn in nurseries. Nurses have become almost as specialized as physicians.

In most larger hospitals the regular nursing staff includes the director of nursing, the nursing supervisor, the head nurse, the floor or staff nurses, the licensed practical nurses (LPNs), the nursing assistants, and the aides. As you move from the beginning to the end of that list, you move down the ladder of authority toward more menial duties.

The director of nursing, the nursing supervisor, the head nurse, and the staff nurses are generally all registered nurses (RNs). They have completed one of several types of nursing training programs. The higher their position in the hospital, the more likely it is that they have a college degree, or even a master's degree. All RNs take a state examination and are licensed by the state to practice nursing. They are all required to have some fundamental understanding of most diseases and of how to observe and manage patients. "RN" appears on the name plate of all registered nurses, male and female.

The director of nursing is the highest nursing authority in the hospital. She is responsible for hiring and firing and reviewing the conduct of the entire nursing staff. She generally works closely with the hospital administrator, the medical director, and the hospital board to set policies and evaluate nursing performance.

Directly under her in power, authority, and responsibility are the nursing supervisors; they are in charge of major nursing areas. These individuals may work with the head nurses (usually assigned

to a particular floor) to schedule nursing coverage or move personnel around to meet ever-changing patient needs. More important,
they maintain close contact with floor activities. They don't personally care for patients (although they almost surely did at one
time in their careers), but they personally oversee the nursing
operations on the floors. They troubleshoot, trying to head off
problems before they arise. If you have a serious complaint about
nursing care, if you can't resolve your problems with the regular
floor nurses or the head nurse, the supervisor, who has overall
responsibility for your area, may be a good person to contact. She
can be a valuable ally for the patient-in-need.

The RNs on the floor are the highest full-time authorities
there. At the top is the head nurse. She directs the others, gives out
assignments, checks the performance of her associates and assistants. She may or may not actually spend time with the patient,
depending upon how busy the ward is, how much nursing help
there is, and whether special problems arise.

The other RNs on the floor are called staff or floor nurses.
They handle patient jobs that require some special knowledge:
dispensing medications; making regular patient observations and
recording them in the chart; changing intravenous bottles; adjusting tubes, drains, respirators, and other medical devices. It is their
job to recognize clinical problems and to call the physician when
they occur.

Except in the case of small hospitals that may have limited
nursing personnel, the RNs generally do not take care of making
beds, bringing and emptying bedpans, helping patients to the
bathroom, giving backrubs, turning on the TV, or feeding the
patient. Not that they never do these things. They may on occasion. But, if less trained personnel are available, they are the ones
who take care of these "routine" patient needs. This may seem like
professional snobbery, and to some extent it is. However, there is
also a valid reason. The RNs are skilled individuals, and their time
is much better spent handling problems that require their special
talents. If an RN is busy feeding a patient—a task that almost
anyone can handle—she can't be paying attention to the patient
with a high fever who needs close specialized observation. It stands
to reason that quality patient care calls for the proper use of

nursing skills. For this reason you should understand why the floor nurse calls someone else, a licensed practical nurse or an aide, to feed you. It is possible that she may feel that this is beneath her and "just isn't her job," but her expertise *can* be put to better use. Put yourself in the position of the very sick patient. Would you be pleased if your intravenous bottle ran dry because the nurse was tied up giving your neighbor a bath?

The LPNs are generally graduates of a one-year course. They have some medical knowledge, but considerably less than the RNs. The exception may be the very intelligent LPN who has been around sick patients for a long time and has picked up a good deal by on-the-job experience. LPNs do take state examinations and are licensed to practice nursing within specified bounds. Because their formal training is less extensive, they cannot do all of the things the RN can. They generally do not give injections or intravenous drugs, adjust sophisticated medical devices, or make independent observations of the patient's condition that may require notation in the chart or notification of the physician. They do take the patient's vital signs—temperature, pulse rate, respiration—deliver oral medications to the patient, and assist with many of the personal needs the patient may have. How many of these needs she'll help with and how many she'll delegate to lower echelon people depends on several things: how busy she is, how nice she is, how concerned about her status and prerogatives she is, how many aides and assistants are available.

The lowest level of floor care comes from the nursing aides and assistants. These individuals are trained by the hospital, or occasionally in brief outside courses, to take care of routine, mundane, basic patient needs. They have no medical education or training and have no licenses. The assistants have badges that may say "NA" (nursing assistant), "aide" (nursing aide), or related abbreviations. Nursing assistants feed patients who can't feed themselves. They assist patients in getting out of bed, going to the bathroom, moving on and off of bedpans. They give baths, make beds, and generally help ensure patient comfort and dignity. As we will see in the next chapter, the treatment you'll receive from the aides and all of the other nursing personnel is partly outside your control. But when you understand their feelings and time constraints and call them only when you really need them, communication between you and the nursing staff will generally flow more smoothly.

Besides these nurses who are with you all the time, there are other nursing personnel you should know about. Some of them may never see you, and you may never need them. Some may take care of certain special needs you may have. Some, at the highest levels, may be the ones to go to when others have failed to solve your problems.

Large hospitals in particular may have teaching programs directed toward the staff nurses or a school for new nurses-in-training. The nursing educators may not wear the usual nurses' uniforms and will rarely come in contact with you, the patient. Occasionally one may ask your permission to discuss your problem with some of her students or to share something with them. You don't have to comply if you would rather not. If you are too tired or simply not in the mood, you can politely say so. But if it isn't a great inconvenience, it would be nice for you to accommodate her. After all, we all depend on our nurses and we want them to continue learning. An important lesson that a nurse learns from you may someday save someone else's life.

Students in a registered nursing program are a familiar part of many of our larger hospitals. Their colored (blue or green) uniforms, rather than standard nursing white, makes them stand out. They may be actively involved with your care. In fact, a student nurse may be assigned to you personally. Again, you can reject her if you so desire, but we believe that having a nursing student involved in your care is a real plus. An extra hand from a willing, conscientious nurse-in-training is like having a personal friend to help guide you through your hospital stay. Since she is assigned to only a few patients, she'll have time to devote to you. You'll have a companion, a sounding board, and someone who can help you deal with any difficulties you might encounter.

Many hospitals, especially the larger ones, can provide special nurses to deal with your unique problems. Private-duty nurses are the best-known example. These are either RNs or LPNs who are not regular hospital employees but who free-lance as personal nurses for a particualr patient. Whether or not you or a relative needs a private-duty nurse, either part time or round-the-clock, depends on multiple factors, including how sick you are, how close observation you require, how able you are to care for your own personal needs, and how overworked and overloaded the nurses on the floor are. We will talk more about private-duty nurses in the next chapter.

The hospital may have other specialized nurses on staff to serve your particular needs. If you are about to deliver a baby, you may meet a nurse-midwife. Even if you have a private obstetrician who will actually perform the delivery, nurse-midwives (who are trained to carry out deliveries themselves) may be part of the obstetrical team. The sympathy, understanding, reassurance, hand-holding, and breathing exercises that she can share with you may be a godsend.

You or an elderly relative may have special needs related to your own illness. For example, patients who have had colostomies or ileostomies—operations that necessitate the draining of intestinal contents into a bag attached to the outside of the abdomen—need home-care instruction and psychological support. More and more hospitals have "ostomy" nurses who devote their full professional activity to this challenging task of patient education. They make personal visits to the patient, and they direct them to community resources—there are ostomy clubs in most large cities—for ongoing support at home and a return to what, for most patients, is a life as active and fulfilling as it was before.

Similarly, there are nurses who specialize in instructing diabetics to manage their insulin injections properly; others who deal with tracheostomies; still others who counsel cancer patients, patients with terminal illnesses, people who require hemodialysis (artifical kidney) support, parents of dying children, and the list goes on. All hospitals and all communities cannot provide this range of nursing resources. It depends upon the size of the facility and the area it serves, the demand, the interest of the medical community, and the availability of financial support.

In the next chapter we will explore, in more detail, the various services that you can expect from your hospital. We will try to show you how to make the best and fullest use of those personnel and resources that are available.

8

You and the Nurses: Achieving a More Effective Relationship

Many patients' natural inclination is to change their personalities when they enter the hospital. Some become utterly cowed, helpless, passive; others become hostile, demanding, aggressive. These very normal human reactions give those who care for you a false, often negative picture.

To a great extent these responses to illness and hospitalization result from the temporary alteration of the self-image we have so carefully crafted throughout our lifetimes. Now ill, hospitalized, and dependent upon an unfamiliar environment for our survival, we see our self-images diminished.

Then too, hospital personnel sometimes deal with their charges in a manner that encourges either total submission or out-and-out rebellion. A few years ago an intelligent attorney friend of ours was hospitalized for some routine studies. He had discussed the protocol with his physician, and he knew, without question, that he was to be off all medication. The accuracy of the upcoming studies depended upon it. On the second evening of his hospital stay a young nurse arrived with a cup of pink and green tablets, at least ten in all.

"Swallow these down like a good little boy," she said in a singsong, patronizing manner.

Our friend overlooked her impertinence, but he gently refused to take the pills since he knew there was an error.

"Now, now," the nurse went on, "just a little bitsy bit of water will make them go down just fine. No reason to be afraid of a few pills."

Our friend's patience ended, and he responded as any normal adult would and should, "Look, young lady. I would appreciate being addressed with a reasonable degree of respect. Also, I know that I am not to take any medications; you can verify this by calling my physician or checking my order sheet. Until this is done, I will not take those pills."

Unruffled and still unaware of her condescending attitude, the nurse shuffled out of the room muttering, "Some patients are such children." A few minutes later she returned, this time obviously embarrassed." I'm terribly sorry," she said. "It seems I was in the wrong room."

Many patients would have reacted differently to this episode. They would have accepted, without comment, this nurse's approach. They might even have viewed this apparent mother-child relationship as the usual nurse-patient interaction. And most would have taken those pills without question, believing with blind faith that the nurse had to be right. As we move through this chapter we will see that neither blind faith nor acceptance of rude treatment has any place in a hospital setting.

Hospital rules and regulations further add to the weakening of self-esteem. Not since the planned and regulated days of summer camp have most adults had to tolerate the strict, often arbitrary, rules of the hospital: lights out at a certain time, smoking only in designated areas, phone calls only at specified times of the day, visitors during limited hours, only one or two visitors to a patient, a minimal number of personal belongings allowed. Fortunately, as hospitals are becoming more and more cognizant of and responsive to patients' concerns and needs, many of these rules are being modified to reflect true safety and health requirements rather than the whims of hospital administrators.

Some of the annoyances you encounter in the hospital are unavoidable and unalterable. There are policies which are basic to hospital safety. Certain protocols and procedures need to be followed even if, at times, they seem superfluous. For example, patients frequently complain about being awakened in the middle of the night to have their blood pressure, pulse, and respiration checked: seemingly an inappropriate interference with the healthful benefits of a good night's sleep. Yet, reasonably close supervision and monitoring may be vital to your welfare, even a check at 4:00 A.M. On the other hand, being awakened at midnight to be given an optional sleeping pill is utterly ludicrous. No patient has to check his common sense at the door. You have the right to balk at inane intrusions like these. By talking to your physician or the head nurse on the floor, you can eliminate these needless inconveniences.

c⅜↝

HOW TO INCREASE YOUR COMFORT AND SAFETY

Be yourself. Understand that times like these are hard on everyone's self-image. You need not feel guilty about a natural, but disturbing, sense of helplessness. You should consciously strive to overcome this by relaxing and behaving with a normal degree of assertiveness and inquisitiveness. Be sure you learn your plan of treatment from your physician. Have him explain, in detail, what diet you'll be getting, what drugs you'll be given, what tests or special studies are planned, what activity you are permitted. An informed patient is both happier and safer. Furthermore, the fact that you know and care about what's going on indicates to everybody that you haven't given up your individuality, intelligence, or common sense.

Deal with all of the hospital personnel as equals, as other human beings, as individuals who have some responsibility for your welfare, but not as personal servants or godlike protectors. This approach will help you to maintain a proper perspective and, at the same time, develop good rapport.

If you are well enough and feel up to it, it helps to find out who's who and who does what. We discussed this in Chapter 7.

Addressing the nurses by their names adds a personal touch. If you are physically able to extend yourself, treat the nurses with respect, not reverence; it will stimulate a reciprocal response on their part. If, however, you are very uncomfortable, you also have the right to expect that the personnel will forgive your dispensing with these amenities and still be supportive. Anything less should, at the appropriate time, bring a complaint from you or your family. We will explain later how this is done.

Try to do as much for yourself as you are physically able and as your doctor permits. Most patients need regular rest or have scheduled tests which necessitate their staying in standard hospital garb—pajamas or nightgown and bathrobe. But there comes a time for many patients—a few days before discharge for example—when they are up most of the time and are physically able to dress. As soon as you comfortably can, get dressed. It boosts your sense of well-being and helps restore your self-image from patient to healthy person.

The same applies to simple personal tasks. No one expects an individual just out of the operating room to jump out of bed and into the bathroom. As long as you need help getting water, eating, getting to the bathroom or on and off of the bedpan, having reading materials brought to you, or answering the telephone, you can properly expect to be given the help you need. But, gradually, as your condition permits, you should begin to do more and more of these things for yourself. The nurses appreciate it when patients who are able to, help themselves. It permits them to spend more time taking care of the more needy. In addition, a return to self-sufficiency is therapeutic for you—it is a big step toward returning home.

All health care personnel appreciate signs of gratitude. A simple, but sincere, "thank-you" is often enough. Candy, cookies, fruit, or a bouquet of flowers placed at the nursing station by one of your relatives expresses special appreciation for a job well done. These tokens are appreciated at any time, but most people wait until the day they leave. Actually, if they are given during your hospital stay, they can reward you with extra considerations beyond the routine. Perhaps this smacks of bribery to carry out expected duties. Maybe so, but the reality is that health care personnel, like most other people, respond to a thoughtful gift or a personal thank-you for a job that is mentally and physically demanding.

HOW TO ASSESS YOUR NEEDS REALISTICALLY

One of the largest problem areas in patient-hospital relations is the discrepancy between the patient's and the nurses' perception of what he needs. To cite some examples: when you are suffering, you want relief from pain immediately. On the other hand, a nurse, facing a life-threatening emergency and knowing that your pain is difficult but not life threatening, will treat the emergency situation first. Generally, in a well-staffed hospital, this conflict should not arise too often, and most patients may expect a reasonably fast response to a request for pain relief. In hospitals that have a shortage of staff, or particularly at night, delays are somewhat more common. In situations like these, where unavoidable circumstances may clash with your expectations, putting the situation into perspective may help to relieve your tension. As a general guideline, we suggest that you discuss your concerns with the staff nurse in charge of your care. Find out why your pain shot took longer to arrive than you believed reasonable. If the answer is unsatisfactory or if you still have doubt or some resentment, you can discuss the matter further with other hospital authorities. We will tell you with whom and how in a later section.

There are countless other examples of the discrepancy between the patient's perception of his needs and the response of the nurses. Some of the more common are your need to sleep versus the need to check your status throughout the night; your desire for a warm bedpan versus the problem of warming them; your desire for water and ice replenishment at once; your wish to have delectable hot food rather than bland, cool usual hospital fare; your belief, and a common patient misconception, that all wounds need to be dressed in a meticulous sterile fashion (wounds themselves are not sterile); your desire for peace and quiet dampened by the all-night movement of people and the clatter of equipment.

Many of these differences and patient annoyances simply

cannot be eliminated. Perhaps, in a perfect, patient-directed hospital utopia they would be, but in the real world of hospital activity and hospital personalities they are not. Some of these concerns can be allayed if you actively communicate with the nurses or your physician. Some you will come to understand better; others, if truly serious or dangerous, will be rectified. To help you understand what you can properly expect from the hospital personnel, let's try to separate the more common, trivial patient complaints from the more serious deficiencies.

Handling Your Minor Complaints

If your food is too cold, if your pain shot took five minutes longer to arrive than you anticipated, if you were left on the bedpan for a few extra minutes, if an aide was somewhat curt, if a physician appeared disheveled, the appropriate response is a simple comment. Minor problems like these interfere with your comfort or sensibilities, but not your physical welfare. A quiet discussion with the right people can help solve these grievances. The ideal sounding board, now available in many hospitals, is the patient representative, or ombudsman, or in some cases, a member of the social service department. Many hospitals now assign such a person to each patient. He or she is your personal agent, your liaison with the hospital staff. It is his or her job to do everything possible to make you comfortable and happy. They know whom to contact on the medical or nursing staff on your behalf to help ameliorate these problems or, at least, to help you understand the reasons for them.

Many hospitals are now distributing admission manuals to patients that offer a number of suggestions, including how and to whom to direct various complaints. If your hospital gives you one of these, review it and use it as a guide. If there is no ombudsman, social worker, or patient representative and you have no printed guide, the staff nurse is the first to contact with your grievance. Speak to the daytime nurse whom you see day after day and whom you know the best. Weekenders or evening nurses are often less in touch with the hospital hierarchy and less able to help. Discuss your concerns calmly, adultly, rationally, and without rancor. You will generally find that the staff nurse is willing to listen and to offer useful advice or to assist in correcting problems.

The staff nurse herself may be the subject of your dissatisfaction. Even then, communicating your concerns to her may improve the situation. She may not even be aware of the fact that you are distressed or that she is doing something that bothers you. If that fails, the next line of authority is the head nurse on the floor. You are entitled to confer with the head nurse and to discuss your problems with her. Generally you will have to go no further. The head nurse wants to maintain patient harmony. She has a very personal interest in keeping her floor comfortable for both occupants and employees.

Handling Your Major Complaints

What if you come across a situation that seriously threatens your well-being or that of your loved one? Let's take a look at some possibilities, first by offering some insights to help you evaluate the quality of nursing care.

The quality of nursing care depends upon the nurse-to-patient ratio—there may simply not be enough nurses or they may be impossibly overworked—and the professional competency of the nurses. Nursing education alone does not automatically imply top-notch training, skill, or concern about patients. What's more, the training of different level nurses is quite variable and their relative expertise reflects this (we discussed the various types of nurses in the previous chapter).

Certain basic parameters form the underpinnings of good nursing care. Here are a few guidelines to help you judge the quality of care you or a relative is receiving:

• Are the nurses attentive? Do they observe you every few hours if you are not seriously ill? For someone who is very ill, are they coming by at shorter intervals—every fifteen minutes or so—depending upon the patient's status?

• Do they answer calls promptly? They may not be able to handle the request immediately, but they should respond verbally to a call at once, either by coming to your room or by using the intercom (if the hospital has them). If they don't do this, they can't know whether your request is urgent or routine.

• Do they take the time to ask important questions: "Any changes in your condition?" "Any pain?" "New complaints?" "How does the cast feel?"

• Do they spend a few minutes with you, or do they seem impossibly rushed and unable to hear you out?

• Do they seem to have an interest in you and your problems? Every nurse can't be a Florence Nightingale, but a certain degree of concern and compassion are prerequisites to quality nursing care.

• Does the nurse call your doctor if an untoward change occurs or if you request that your doctor be called?

• Is there some continuity in nursing care—one or two of the same faces per shift? Replacement nurses are necessary, but some hospitals move nurses from place to place excessively or regularly use part-timers to service their floors. Some continuity of nursing care is important. The nurses get to know you and your problem and can tell if something has changed or is amiss.

• Are the nurses properly skilled and specialized to deal with your particular problem? Many nurses cannot interpret an electrocardiogram, but nurses who work in a coronary care unit must be able to. It takes special skills beyond general nursing training to manage sick children, intensive care problems, patients in traction, women in labor, or psychiatric problems.

If you can't give positive replies to each of these questions, there may be serious nursing care deficiencies. These potentially dangerous shortcomings cannot be ignored. Don't wait for a catastrophe. Notify your physician. Your doctor is ultimately responsible for your welfare. He wants his orders to be carried out properly, and he must intervene actively if nursing errors jeopardize your well-being.

Sometimes a move to another section of the hospital will afford better care—the quality of the nursing staff often varies quite markedly from floor to floor. Some additional assistance from a private-duty nurse may be beneficial in your particular case. You may even consider a transfer to another hospital if the nursing deficiencies are intolerable and unsafe. Fortunately, such dramatic remedies are rarely necessary. With proper input from you, even major nursing care problems are usually correctable.

HOW YOU CAN HELP PATIENTS WITH SPECIAL-CARE NEEDS

Elderly Patients

Elderly patients often have special needs, eccentricities, or routines that the nurses, if aware of them, could accommodate. These special needs can be very important to an elderly patient. The nurses are grateful to learn about them because often these simple things can make the difference between a confused, disoriented patient and a reasonably comfortable, well-adjusted one. Examples might include: prune juice each morning and evening (or a favorite laxative)—many patients, young as well as old, are troubled by a disruption of their usual bowel habits; a morning newspaper (as long as it's not delivered at 6:00 A.M. by a vendor shouting "NEWSPAPER!"; one of us recently faced this during an unpleasant five-day hospital stay); a night light; morning visits from a clergyman; milk at a certain hour; a daily vitamin; and music to sleep by. If you let the nurses know of these habits, preferably on admission when the history is obtained, this can smooth the adjustment of your elderly friend or relative. The more homelike the atmosphere, the easier the transition to hospital life.

Handicapped Patients

A patient may have physical or mental handicaps which, while relevant to his ability to help himself, may not be directly related to his current health problem. Your eighty-year-old grandmother may be in the hospital for treatment of pneumonia, but she may also be paralyzed on the left side from an earlier stroke, hard-of-hearing, and partially senile. The nurses directly responsible for her care will know of her general health problems. Others who may have occasional contact with her will not. Dietary personnel, housekeepers, X-ray technicians, laboratory workers, transport staff, various therapists, and even maintenance people may need to communicate with her. We've witnessed numerous embarrassing episodes that occurred because these individuals were unaware of the patient's limitations. Once one of us was examining a patient. In the next bed lay an elderly gentleman, obviously hard-of-hearing and somewhat senile. In popped the food-service woman, plunked his food down, and without waiting for a reply announced, "Lunch is here." If I hadn't informed an aide that the man's food had arrived and he needed help eating, the meal would have been untouched until the lady from the food service returned to collect the tray.

How best to handle this kind of problem depends on the individual involved, how frequently visitors will be present, and whether or not the expense of special nursing care makes that a viable option. Private-duty nurses can help individuals like these. The problem is that this service is very costly (we will discuss this in the next section). If relatives or friends will be spending a great deal of time with the patient, they can actively assist the bedridden individual. Another very effective method that is frequently employed is to attach a sign to the patient's bed noting his or her disability. For some patients, we realize, this can be embarrassing. For this reason, if they can understand, they should be consulted first.

PRIVATE-DUTY NURSES

Private-duty nurses are hired by patients as their personal attendants. The hospital may have a list of available nurses, or the patient or his family can deal with an agency or with nurses who advertise their services. Listings are available in the telephone directory. Better yet, the best source is a personal referral from your doctor, a friend, or relative. This offers the advantage of prescreening.

Some health insurance policies pay for private-duty nurses. Many do not, and their services are quite expensive. Round-the-clock RNs cost approximately two thousand dollars per week. The fee for an LPN or an aide is commensurately less, seven hundred to fifteen hundred dollars per week. Thus, it is often the well-to-do patients who employ them, particularly for prolonged periods.

Whether or not a private-duty nurse is right for you depends upon several factors: the kind of care you need, the quality and adequacy of the hospital nursing staff, and how well you can prescreen the private-duty nurse.

If you are in a large, well-staffed hospital and you have a specialized health care problem, private-duty nurses may be more harmful than helpful. Because a private-duty nurse may come from any walk of nursing life, it is unlikely that she will have special expertise in your particular problem. If you have just had an operation, it is more likely that the floor nurses are more attuned to postoperative problems than the private nurse would be. If your child is hospitalized with pneumonia, the hospital-based nurses are probably familiar with pediatric patients. The private-duty nurse may not be. Specialty problems, intensive care, monitoring of serious injuries or illnesses are, therefore, generally better handled by the hospital staff. But doesn't the private nurse merely complement the hospital staff? Does her presence eliminate regular hospital nursing care? To a certain degree it does. Not by hospital design, but in actual practice, once a private nurse appears, the regular floor nurses pay less attention to the patient. They reason that the patient has a nurse. The patient then becomes very dependent on the expertise—which is highly variable—of the private-duty nurse. In general it is safer to rely on hourly observations by a skilled, specialized RN than on constant observation by a potentially less skilled private nurse. Please understand, not all private-duty nurses are unskilled. Some are superb. But if you are assigned one, or you choose one at random, you are dealing with an unknown. Unless you have been assured— either by your doctor or friends—that the particular nurse is qualified to handle your problem, you take a chance.

Private-duty nurses are invaluable in certain situations. In understaffed hospitals, where the regular floor nurses can't attend all of their patients adequately, an ever-present helping hand is a valuable asset. If you have had minor surgery, are not terribly ill (therefore don't require superskilled nursing observation), but simply need an extra pair of hands for a few days, a private nurse can be a real blessing. One exceptional private-duty nurse we know insists that her most important function is "to fight for her patients, to make them do what they should do but are afraid to do, and to provide a certain continuity of nursing care that may not be possible with a more frequently changing hospital staff." Other patients who are in need of physical assistance can benefit immeasurably from the help of a private-duty nurse. Helping the now-stabilized stroke victim to get back on his feet, assisting a child in a full-body cast to get around, providing comfort and a feeling of security for a temporarily sightless man whose patched eyes are recovering from recent surgery are all useful services that private-duty nurses can provide. They offer extra hands, eyes, ears, and legs for those who need them.

9

The Physician Staff
and How It Affects You Personally

The levels of medical authority in a hospital are as distinct as the chain of command in a Marine Corps unit. There is a significant difference however. In a hospital, though the respective roles and ranks of various physicians are clearly delineated, the exercise of power and the use of discipline is, at present, less formalized than it is in the military environment. But that is changing rapidly.

Only a few years ago hospitals had almost no control over, and relatively little interest in, the conduct of their physician staff. Now the pressures of federal regulations, surveillance by the Joint Commission on Accreditation of Hospitals (JCAH), and new court decisions in liability lawsuits have stimulated sweeping changes. Certain sections of the country, and certain types of small physician-run hospitals, lag behind, but the majority of American hospitals have responded to these new pressures by tightening their supervision and control over their physicians. They have (often reluctantly) accepted the inescapable fact that the hospital, as a service facility, is more than a collection of rooms where independent physicians place their patients. It is a social institution endowed with a profound public trust. It has a responsibility to see to it that the quality of medical care offered by its nurses and its physicians meets certain reasonable standards.

⚜

HOW TO UNDERSTAND THE CHAIN OF COMMAND AND WHY IT IS IMPORTANT TO YOU

There are two levels of medical command in the hospital: the first is administrative and is responsible for physician surveillance and discipline; the second is directly responsible to you, the patient. Since the latter is your medical care team, we will dwell on this chain of command at some length later in this chapter. The first, the administrative hierarchy, is only important to you if you want to lodge a major complaint, or if you are simply curious about the inner workings of the medical staff. We will deal, very briefly, with this aspect of the hospital structure.

The board of directors are generally prominent nonphysician members of the community. They have the ultimate responsibility for the people who use the hospital. They set hospital policies and try to make the hospital responsive to community needs.

The *hospital administrator* is a nonphysician. He is in charge of both financial and administrative matters. Essentially he is like the company president who, along with many advisers and directors, implements hospital procedures and practices. He works closely with the *medical director or chief of medical staff* who is a physician-administrator. This individual has a medical background and, therefore, serves as the liaison and interface among the physician staff, the hospital board, and the hospital administrator. The medical director is a nonpracticing physician. He is a full-time administrator. Many smaller hospitals have no such individual on staff.

Some hospitals have a *chief of the medical staff* instead of a medical director. He or she is a practicing physician, and in many smaller hospitals that cannot afford a full-time medical director, the chief of staff assumes all of the director's functions. The chief of staff is the spokesperson for the medical community. If the doctors feel that new policies, equipment, specialists, or services are needed, he is the one who transmits the message to the administrator and the board of directors.

In a hospital that is divided into various departments, one member of each department is designated as "chief." He may be elected or appointed. The *chief of a department* is charged with developing departmental rules, establishing guidelines for staff privileges in that department, conducting educational and business meetings, and implementing sound teaching programs for physicians-in-training and students (if the hospital has them).

The *attending staff physician* is the individual who is directly responsible for patient care. His office may be in the hospital; usually he will have a private office outside. The *attending staff physicians* are all of the members of the hospital staff who have admitting privileges. Your doctor, if he admits you to the hospital, is on the attending staff. An attending staff physician may be the department chief or simply a member of the department. To become an active staff physician, the doctor must present required credentials and recommendations and, today more and more, must demonstrate a continued level of competency, proficiency, and evidence of some participation in continuing medical education courses.

HOW TO MAKE SURE A COMPLAINT COUNTS

The board of directors and the hospital administrators are vitally concerned with community support. If you or other members of the community have major complaints about the hospital— the quality of the emergency department, the lack of certain specialists, dangerous physical conditions—a phone call or letter to the administrator and chairman of the board is the surest conduit to affirmative action. On the other hand, if you are a patient in the hospital and have complaints about nursing care, the quality of food, or physician errors, a plea to the board is too slow to help you. To iron out problems like these you must deal with the chain of nursing command (outlined in Chapter 8), or the physician hierarchy presented in this chapter.

The Professional Hierarchy

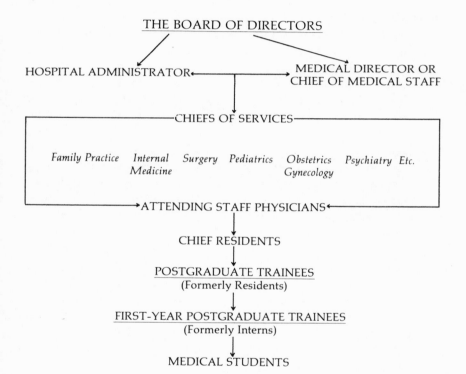

THE BOARD OF DIRECTORS

HOSPITAL ADMINISTRATOR

MEDICAL DIRECTOR OR
CHIEF OF MEDICAL STAFF

CHIEFS OF SERVICES

Family Practice   *Internal* *Surgery* *Pediatrics* *Obstetrics* *Psychiatry* *Etc.*
Medicine   *Gynecology*

ATTENDING STAFF PHYSICIANS

CHIEF RESIDENTS

POSTGRADUATE TRAINEES
(Formerly Residents)

FIRST-YEAR POSTGRADUATE TRAINEES
(Formerly Interns)

MEDICAL STUDENTS

⟨⟩

PHYSICIANS AND THE NONTEACHING HOSPITAL

Admittance to a hospital is arranged by your doctor. No one gets in without one. In fact, you may have a whole contingent of doctors who are, in some way, responsible for your care. As hospitals become increasingly complex, large, and sophisticated, the medical hierarchy expands upward and outward in a confusing arborization. Certain equal members of this medical tree may supplement the services of your personal physician. Others, below him in authority and training, may help him to manage your ongoing medical needs. To help you understand who is who, who does what, and whom to call for help in this sometimes bewildering environment, we will begin with the simplest setting—the small nonteaching hospital. Here your private physician is your primary medical care provider. We will consider the more complex teaching hospital later. There the sheer mass of medical students, physicians-in-training, and consultants can be utterly perplexing.

In the small community hospital your doctor admits you and cares for you. He or she may be a family practitioner, an internist, a pediatrician (if your child is the patient), a surgeon (if an operation is planned). Elective admissions—those that are planned weeks in advance—are arranged by your physician. You are admitted to "his service." This is simply the term that is commonly used to refer to patients under his care. You may be asked, whose service are you on? instead of who is your doctor?

If an emergency situation arises and you have a private physician, he may see you in his office, meet you in the emergency department and admit you himself, or he may refer you to the relevant specialist for in-hospital care. For example, it is unlikely that you have a personal general surgeon or orthopedic surgeon unless you have been the unfortunate victim of previous surgical or orthopedic problems. If you have no favorite surgeon, your general physician will refer you to a specialist who can care for your urgent surgical needs. This surgeon, then, becomes your attending physician.

How to Proceed If You Don't Have a Family Physician

What do you do if you're new to an area, passing through a remote town, or vacationing away from home and a crisis arises—acute appendicitis, for instance?

Once you've reached the emergency department of the nearest hospital, the first physician you'll see will be the individual assigned to the emergency room. If he determines that immediate surgery is in order, he'll contact the surgeon on call. If your problem is a medical one—a heart attack, pneumonia, pancreatitis, blood clots, to name a few—you'll be referred to the general practitioner or the internist on call. If you choose to stay in that hospital, or if your condition leaves you no choice, you may not have any control over which surgeon or which medical specialist becomes "your" doctor. There may only be one person on call or one person available. Or else you may have the option to transfer to another hospital (we discussed this in Chapters 1 and 5). Or, if you become dissatisfied, you may later be able to switch physicians at that hospital. We will discuss how in the next chapter.

Your Physician's Responsibilities

You are now in the hospital, either under the care of your longtime doctor, a colleague to whom he referred you, or a completely unfamiliar physician who was assigned to care for you. As your admitting and attending physician, he or she is responsible for coordinating your medical care. He writes orders that convey his wishes to the nurses. These include: how they should observe and monitor your vital functions, what tests they should order, what physical activity you're permitted, and what drugs you are to be given. The physician makes the decisions; the nurses follow his instructions.

Your physician will generally see you at least once a day—more often if your condition is serious or if the nurses call him, occasionally less if you are completely out of danger. In small hospitals frequently the only physicians you'll ever see are your attending doctor, and if he has signed out for an evening or a weekend, his partner, or replacement. This simplifies the chain of medical command. If you have any questions relating to your medical condition, your medication, perceived deficiences in nursing care, your doctor is the one to approach.

It is often helpful to write out all of your questions as you think of them, otherwise they may slip your mind during his usually brief visit. If you have an urgent problem that can't wait for the next day's visit, ask the floor nurse to contact your doctor. Tell her you want to talk to him. He'll either call you or stop by.

The Role of Consultants

If problems arise which lie outside the scope of your physician's training, he may call in specialist consultants. Even most small hospitals have a wide range of specialists—cardiologists, dermatologists, neurologists, various surgeons—on their staffs. Normally your doctor will let you know that Dr. X will be coming to see you.

Consultants most often supplement the care provided by your primary physician. They are his advisors, but they do not usurp his authority. He remains in charge of your case. However, as we will see in the next chapter, there are times when you may be transferred to the consultant's service. For example: you may be admitted by an internist to evaluate your abdominal pain. Two days later a surgical consultant decides that you have appendicitis. He operates and you are now *his* patient. The internist, originally your primary physician, may see you as a consultant, or he may leave the scene entirely if his services are no longer needed.

The only other physicians you may encounter in some small hospitals are house physicians who oversee patients at night and on weekends. Not all hospitals have this kind of coverage. If they don't, all problems are transmitted by phone by the nurse to the attending physician. If they do have a coverage arrangement—and more and more hospitals today do—the house physician may see you first if you need physician attention. After he examines you and assesses your situation, he will then call your attending physician to discuss a plan of action.

The smaller the hospital, the simpler the medical hierarchy. You may see only one physician—your attending, admitting doctor. You may meet one of his associates, who relieves him for an evening, a weekend, or a vacation period. You may come in contact with one or more specialists if your condition warrants broader evaluation. Finally, if the hospital provides coverage doctors, you might encounter another strange face. But the man or woman in charge is clearly visible. He or she is your private physician, the one who admits you to the hospital and coordinates all of your health care. Except in the most unusual circumstances (discussed in the next chapter) you'll know whom to call for help.

THE TEACHING HOSPITAL

To simplify this discussion, let's consider only one type of teaching hospital—the university hospital. In the university hospital the medical personnel include the students, first-year postgraduates (formerly known as interns), more advanced postgraduate trainees (formerly called residents), chief residents, fellows (postgraduate trainees who have completed a residency and are now further subspecializing), faculty staff members, and consultants of every description. Some nonuniversity teaching hospitals don't have this full complement of young doctors—they may not have medical students for example—but if you can understand the medical structure of the university hospital, any other teaching hospital is simple by comparison. The hierarchy will be the same, only the range of medical trainees may be smaller.

The first problem when you enter the university hospital is to identify the leader of your health care team. If your own physician or a physician to whom you are referred is on the university staff, you may be admitted to his service. He has probably examined you in his office; he may or may not carry out another thorough examination; but he will continually review and reevaluate those aspects of your physical examination and laboratory studies that are important to your current health problem. Then, no matter how many subordinates you see every day, your physician is the ultimate arbiter of your treatment. He may not make all of the decisions: routine matters, such as requesting studies, ordering certain medications, carrying out minor procedures, are left to the house staff (the general term used for all physicians-in-training) or, with close supervision, to medical students. As physicians advance in their training, they are given more and more responsibility. The medical student, for example, must have his orders reviewed and countersigned by an M.D. The chief resident, on the other hand, can make many decisions on his own. However, once those decisions become more complex—for example, a planned operation or a very serious study—the staff physician will invariably be involved.

If you have no private physician and enter a university hospital via the emergency department or via a general referral, two things may happen: (1) You may request the services of a particular staff member—someone you know, have heard of, perhaps the chairman of the department, or a professor in the appropriate department. If you choose this route, then you become the private patient of the physician you select (assuming he is willing to accept you as a patient). Then, at the top of your health care team is the attending staff physician whom you have selected or who has been assigned to you. (2) Alternatively, you need not designate a particular staff member as your doctor. Then, you may be designated a "staff patient." This means that the house-staff physicians are your primary care doctors. Invariably, they have faculty supervision—a member of the attending staff is assigned, on a rotating basis, to oversee the house-staff patients.

Understanding the Role of Various Physicians in a Teaching Hospital

Whether you have your own physician or are a "staff patient," you are likely to encounter the following members of the medical team. Medical students are at the lowest end of the health care team. They are still in school and haven't yet received their M.D. degrees. They are not officially doctors: they are training to become doctors. In most medical schools the course of study lasts four years. The majority of your medical student contacts will be with third- and fourth-year students. The first- and second-year students are more involved in classroom studies, but occasionally they appear on the hospital floors for some supervised instruction in patient care.

Normally the medical student assigned to your floor and to you will want to take a medical history and to examine you. You will also be examined by one or more postgraduate trainees and, perhaps, by your attending staff physician. If you strongly object to a student exam, you ought to discuss this with your attending physician or with the hospital personnel prior to being admitted; there may be sections of the hospital where no students are assigned. Hospital policy (quite variable) may permit you to refuse a student exam, or possibly you may have to be transferred elsewhere in the hospital. Some university hospitals insist on student involvement in patient care in exchange for the superior patient care services that they offer.

Some Surprising Advantages of Being Examined by a Medical Student

We, as physicians, frankly welcome examinations by all members of the health care team, including medical students. We wouldn't permit a student to perform surgery or a potentially dangerous procedure, but a simple examination is risk free. Moreover, the student is enthusiastic, wants to do well, and can spend more time with you than anyone else. They say you can always tell a medical-student work-up because it is five pages long, whereas the intern's is a page and a half, the resident's is a half page, and the senior resident or staff man's is one line. Although the medical student is a novice and doesn't know all of the medical nuances or ramifications, he is bright, interested, and often able to pick up key points that others may miss. Surprisingly often the student will point out a critical finding or historical issue that all of the more senior observers overlooked or failed to elicit. Finally, the medical student is a good medical friend. He has time to devote to his patients, and he becomes a valuable ally—a direct conduit to the higher-ups in the medical chain of command.

The medical student examination will always be supplemented by independent history-taking and examinations by more senior members of the health care team. You will surely be questioned and examined by one or more of the postgraduate trainees. The chief resident will probably conduct a more cursory exam, but he will review the findings of those other physicians and will personally evaluate you if there are areas of confusion, uncertainty, or possible shortcomings.

One level above the medical student we have the first-year postgraduate trainee (formerly known as an intern); he *is a doctor*. Many people don't realize this. We frequently hear patients say, "I want to see a doctor, not an intern." He is generally not licensed to practice medicine beyond the confines of the hospital since most states require this year of training before granting licensure. But he is an M.D., a graduate of a medical school. It is likely that a physician at this level will also be assigned to you. He or she will perform an examination (in addition to the student's exam) and will probably write your initial orders. This level trainee is directly responsible for many of your daily health care needs. He may draw your blood (students do this too), start intravenous lines, insert catheters into your bladder, place tubes through your nose into your stomach, or change your dressings. Rest assured; his orders, his plans, his actions are under constant scrutiny by superiors— more advanced trainees and your staff doctor. The first-year postgraduate physician is another valuable member of your health care team. He is readily available when you need him and has immediate access to the more senior physicians.

The more senior trainees are qualified physicians, licensed to practice medicine. Many general practitioners have no more formal training than these second- to sixth-year postgraduate trainees. These members of your team are in training to fine-tune their medical skills or to gain special expertise in a complex medical or surgical specialty.

The composition of your health care team varies from hospital to hospital, floor to floor, service to service (medicine, pediatrics, surgery, orthopedics). It may include a student, a first-year postgraduate physician, a more advanced trainee, and the chief resident. At the very top is the attending staff physician.

To better understand this team approach, assume you have appendicitis. Dr. Jones, staff surgeon, will perform the operation. Dr. Jones will not ask you about childhood diseases or your family health history. He will probably not listen to your heart or look in your ears. The student and postgraduate physicians-in-training will conduct those aspects of your evaluation—the areas not specifically related to the appendicitis. On the other hand, Dr. Jones will surely place his stethoscope on your abdomen and palpate the tender area. And he will review your white blood count value, all important criteria in his diagnosis of appendicitis.

How the "Team" Coordinates Your Care

Medical rounds, once or twice daily, provide the vital link between these individuals and your health care needs. The team visits you and discusses your problems. Then, generally in private, they review your progress, formulate a plan of action, and assign specific responsibilities to each team member. Your attending staff physician may make rounds daily with the team or may accompany the group two or three times weekly. In the interim the chief resident keeps him abreast of your progress and requests advice as necessary.

The university hospital provides a pyramidal system of patient care. At the very top is your private or attending staff physician. He is invested with ultimate authority and responsibility. In the final analysis, all serious decisions, such as operating or not operating or performing a potentially dangerous study, are his to make. You will never find yourself wheeled into the operating room without having discussed this with him. In the unlikely instance that this might happen, *Protest!* Don't agree to surgery or to any major procedures without conferring with the staff physician in charge of your care.

On the other hand, you may be sent for a chest X-ray, some routine blood studies, or other minor tests or procedures without having an official go-ahead from the man at the top. These minor daily procedures can be requested by the junior members of the health care team. There is no reason that your attending physician has to be involved with trivial matters like these.

Special problems outside the expertise of your health care team may bring consultants to your bedside. Consultations may be performed by any of three levels of physicians: postgraduate trainees in the particular specialty; fellows—physicians who have finished several years of postgraduate training and are now subspecializing (in cardiology, gastroenterology, infectious diseases, cardiac surgery, etc.); or fully trained staff members. In general, the more complex your problem, the higher level consultant you'll see. Or a junior member of the consulting team may see you first and then call for help from a more experienced specialist if he has any questions or uncertainties.

In the next chapter we will give you some useful tips on how to deal with these physicians and how to ensure that their efforts and recommendations are properly coordinated.

10

Physician Care
in the Hospital: The Benefits of
Being Aware and Involved

WHO IS YOUR DOCTOR? DO YOU
REALLY KNOW?

By now a loud crash in the living room had become a familiar sound. Once again your seventy-year-old mother had shuffled into the blurred outline of your glass coffee table. Now it was a matter of life and limb. Much as you both regretted it, she had to have that cataract operation.

After reconferring with Dr. Blaire, her ophthalmologist, your mother made an appointment to see her family practitioner, Dr. Levy. She had no significant health problems, but a complete physical examination was precautionary. Moreover, the hospital routinely required a presurgical examination on all patients. Your mother visited Dr. Levy's office one week prior to her planned admission date. He gave her a thorough examination and told her she was ready for surgery. Dr. Levy could have examined her in the hospital (preoperative examinations are often done that way), but there are advantages to the office exam: it can shorten the hospital stay by a day or two, and it can head off a wasted admission should an abnormal finding necessitate postponing the operation.

On March 20, Dr. Blaire admitted your mother to the community hospital. There were no physicians-in-training in this small hospital. Your mother was on Dr. Blaire's service, and he alone was responsible for her medical supervision.

So far your mother's story seems fairly typical. A doctor, her own ophthalmologist, put her in the hospital. She, her family, and the nurses knew who that doctor was. You would assume that most people, except those who are unconscious or very confused, know their doctor. However, strange things can happen to patients in hospitals.

As physical problems change, doctors may also change. When a simple problem erupts into a multisystem breakdown, a new medical team may be summoned, new physicians may take control—at times so frequently and so rapidly that the patient himself has no idea who is in command. Take your mother's case. Two days after the operation, just when a smooth recovery seemed inevitable, her heart suddenly began to beat erratically. Promptly, an alert nurse called her physician, Dr. Blaire. He arrived at her bedside within a half hour. Since he knew little about managing malfunctioning hearts, he called in Dr. Levy, the family practitioner. Dr. Levy gave your mother a well-chosen drug which stabilized her heartbeat. In a brief conference which followed, both doctors agreed that a change in command would be in your mother's best interest. Dr. Levy would take charge.

Since your mother's heart problem was potentially more treacherous and life threatening than her recent eye surgery, she would now be on Dr. Levy's service. Dr. Blaire would examine her eye daily, but Dr. Levy was now the physician-of-record. He would handle any calls from the nurses and would, in turn, watch your mother closely.

The nurses were told of the change. The doctor's name on her chart was changed from Blaire to Levy. Your mother stayed in the same room. Nobody, however, remembered to tell you or your mother about the change of doctors.

The first you learned of this change in command was two days later when you asked the nurse to call Dr. Blaire to order something for your mother's constipation. "Dr. Blaire? Your mother's not on his service now. Dr. Levy is the physician in charge," was the reply. How could a change as important as that have taken place without your consent or participation? Even worse, when you confronted your mother with the news, she was as surprised as you were.

The next day you let Dr. Levy know, with no pretext of disguising your annoyance, what you thought of these interdoctor arrangements. He apparently got your message, for eight hours later when your mother's cardiac rhythm became more erratic, he simultaneously summoned Dr. Bennett, a consultant cardiologist, *and you*. Together, all three of you and your mother concurred that a transfer to Dr. Bennett's care in the coronary care unit was in order.

Now Dr. Levy was gone from the scene entirely. In this case (quite variable from situation to situation) he fully relinquished his role. His function was usurped by someone more specialized. Dr. Blaire, on the other hand, continued seeing your mother daily, making sure that her eye steadily healed.

Your mother's simple relationship with Dr. Blaire—her only physician—became complicated by two switches: first to Dr. Levy, then to Dr. Bennett. But compared with the game of musical doctors that can occur, her three-doctor move was simple indeed.

She was fortunate to have had only two organs in jeopardy— her eye and her heart—keeping the number of physicians to a manageable level. At times, widespread and diverse complications may call forth a confusing array of medical practitioners.

There often seems to be little rhyme or reason to patterns of consultations and transfers. They vary from hospital to hospital, doctor to doctor, and patient to patient. A consultant in a particular field might merely act as an adviser to the admitting physician, or he may take over primary care responsibility. There are no written guidelines or official rules to tell the consultant when he is just a consultant and when he should become *the doctor*. The one situation in which a formal transfer almost always occurs is when a patient, admitted by a nonsurgeon, develops a surgical problem and needs immediate surgery. Then the surgeon almost invariably takes over the patient's care. But when a neurologist, a pulmonary specialist, a kidney expert, or a cardiologist is asked to help out the internist or family practitioner, he will most often just help out, but he may take over. The decision is made by mutual consent of the physicians (and, hopefully, the patient—although, as we have seen, that isn't always so). They decide whose clinical expertise is most urgently and intensely required. So, if a complication or a diagnostic dilemma arises and you are seen by one or more consultants, one of two things may happen: you may remain under the care of your admitting physician with the additional guidance of the consultants, or you may be transferred to the care of a specialist, in which case you may or may not see your admitting physician again during your hospital stay.

Unfortunately, as happened in your mother's case, the patient may be the last to know about a transfer: which doctor is a consultant and which is really the main manager. Surprisingly, and potentially dangerous, on occasion the nurses and even the doctors themselves don't know. Communications can break down and the patient may be left with no doctor in charge.

A few years ago one of us came across a patient who had been lost for a week. And this was in a major university hospital. The patient was originally on a surgical service because of a suspected appendicitis. In two days, without surgery, he improved, and the surgical resident requested a consultation with an internal medicine resident.

The new diagnosis was either an ulcer or pancreatitis, conditions not requiring immediate surgery. Then the misunderstanding occurred. Believing that the patient's transfer had been okayed, the surgical resident sent him, with a set of new nurses' orders, to the medical floor. However the medical resident, feeling that the patient should stay on the surgical service, had not authorized any transfer.

The nurses on the medical floor assumed that the medical resident realized that the new arrival was his responsibility. Two days later the interns and the residents changed rotations, as they do every month or two, and a new group came onto the floor. The lost patient remained unattended.

Meanwhile the patient thought it was rather strange that he hadn't seen a doctor for several days, but by that time he was much better. Orders had been written and the nurses gave him what he needed and wanted. Presumably he was satisfied with this "benign neglect." Finally, after six days, he spoke up and asked one of the nurses where his doctor was and when he was going home. Only then did they realize that no physician had seen this patient or had any knowledge of his existence. He was literally a patient without a doctor. The error was quickly rectified, and the hospital changed its transfer system so that a mistake like that could never happen again.

Fortunately that man wasn't very sick. He didn't need medical care, and he got better without a physician-in-charge. Of course, being at home would have been far less expensive.

We have seen other cases—mostly in the context of medical malpractice suits—where confusion about lines of responsibility has culminated in serious patient injury or death.

A child was hospitalized with a severe asthmatic attack. The general practitioner, not able to control the situation, called a pediatrician for help. He came in, and together they stabilized the four-year-old girl. The pediatrician believed that his role was clear: he was the consultant, not the primary physician. The general practitioner was certain that he had relinquished the care of the child and had turned her over to the pediatrician. Each believed that the other had written medication orders and monitoring instructions for the nurses to follow. In fact, neither had entered any instructions in the chart. Consequently the child did not receive medications that she urgently needed; nor did she get the close nursing supervision that her precarious condition required.

Four hours later, during a routine check, the child was found to be blue and gasping for air. Emergency resuscitation by a nearby in-house-physician saved the child's life, but many minutes of oxygen deprivation took its toll. The child's brain was severely damaged.

In the malpractice suit that followed the facts came out: each physician had assumed that the other was in charge. Both doctors were found to be negligent for failing to clarify their responsibilities. The hospital, too, was held responsible because it had not promulgated a checks-and-balance system to prevent this kind of error. Again, the hospital changed its policy, unfortunately in the wake of a permanently injured child.

Patients who are admitted from emergency departments to the service of a private physician can suffer from inattention and uncertain leadership. Here's another example of a malpractice suit, in this case naming an emergency department physician, a hospital, and a private gynecologist.

A young woman was hospitalized by the emergency department physician because of pelvic pain and a high fever. His diagnosis: an infection of the tubes and ovaries. He couldn't locate Dr. Benson, the gynecologist-on-call, so he initiated treatment, wrote admission orders, and placed this young woman on Dr. Benson's service. He reasoned that she would be all right through the night and that Dr. Benson would learn about the admission the next day. However the emergency department physician had not charted a proper course for observation or treatment. He had requested checks every four hours by the nurses, but this woman needed much closer monitoring than that. Moreover, he had not ordered any antibiotics to combat her infection.

At 4:00 A.M., the first four-hour-check, the girl was found to be terribly ill. The nurses tried to contact Dr. Benson, who still wasn't home. After two hours of abortive attempts, they finally found another surgeon to evaluate this woman. He operated at once, but she succumbed to massive peritonitis.

At the trial all three—the hospital, the emergency physician, and Dr. Benson—were found negligent. Dr. Benson had never seen this woman in his life; but she was admitted to his service, and he was on call that night. His was a bizarre case of malpractice by proxy. The emergency department physician was negligent for admitting her without talking to the appointed attending physician (when he should have called someone else) and for writing poor orders. The hospital was guilty too, for permitting a patient to be admitted without formal notification of the attending physician and for accepting orders from someone other than the doctor of record.

Sick patients can also, occasionally, get lost in the shuffle or suffer from inattention when the primary physician goes off duty. He may simply go out for the evening, away for a weekend, or on vacation for a month. In general, conscientious physicians will discuss these plans with their patients and will arrange for competent coverage. They will also communicate with the new physician and will be certain that his replacement knows just what's happening and what to expect with each patient. But, as you can easily imagine, this kind of interdoctor communication and delegation of responsibility can be a weak link in patient care. The new physician can't possibly know his temporary charges as well as the principal physician can. Or the primary physician may inadvertently fail to provide full information. How comforting it would be if we could faithfully assume that our doctors and nurses are always in full control and flawless. We would like to leave the details to them and lie back and relax with complete confidence that knowledgeable people are in charge and errors won't occur. Most of the time this assumption holds true.

HOW TO MAKE SURE THAT YOUR MEDICAL CARE IS WELL COORDINATED

Usually you know who the doctor-in-charge is and so do the nursing personnel and the physician himself. But, as we have seen, slip-ups occur. Our advice: take charge. Check with both your physician and the nurses to be certain that everyone knows who is responsible for your care and that everyone comes up with the same answer.

When consultants arrive to evaluate specific problems, ask them and your doctor what their roles are. Are they advisers to your physician, or does he expect one of them to be taking over? Be sure that your physician and the consultants have the same understanding. For example, if a cardiologist is called in to evaluate your heart problem, ask him how he will interrelate with your original doctor. Then ask your physician. If the cardiologist tells you that he is merely a consultant but your own doctor tells you that the cardiologist is the new captain of your ship, you have found a potentially serious discrepancy that needs to be ironed out. Since it's your health that can suffer if communications go awry, you must, for your own protection, be certain that the entire medical team is well coordinated.

What if you are admitted directly from the emergency department? You never saw your admitting physician—either your private doctor or someone assigned to your care. Ask the nurses whether they, themselves, notified the doctor who will be caring for you that you are there. Ask them whether they discussed your problem with him and whether he personally provided orders for you. If the emergency department physician wrote the orders, was your doctor at least informed? Did he concur with the treatment plan? As you can see, there is a remote but real danger when your admission is initiated by the emergency department personnel. "Your" doctor may not know he's "your" doctor. In fact, he may not even be in town. An inquiry from you can eliminate this kind of error.

If your physician tells you that he is leaving you in the hands of an associate, request a visit from the new physician. It is ideal, but not always practical or possible, for both doctors to come together. Whether or not a joint visit is necessary depends on how sick you are and how much attention you are likely to need. Obviously, the more serious or pressing your needs, the more certain you must be that the new doctor is well oriented.

⊱✣⊰

HOW TO KNOW WHOM TO TALK TO WHEN YOUR CARE IS A TEAM APPROACH

In university hospitals and other institutions with physicians-in-training, knowing who's in charge may be very confusing indeed. We've gone through the makeup of the health care team in the previous chapter. We've also seen that the parade of potential consultant after consultant can make you reel in utter confusion. There are several tricks that can make life much easier for you. First, be aware of the fact that the man at the top—the private attending physician or the chief of your service—may not see you every day and may not be as accessible as some of the more junior members of the health care team. If the "boss" isn't always available, it is helpful for you to identify a team member whom you can use as your personal coordinator. This may be the chief resident or one of the junior physicians-in-training who visits you on rounds. The choice may be a very natural one; for example, you may find that a first-year postgraduate trainee is always on the floor and quite willing to stop by and discuss your problems with you. The person you select doesn't necessarily have to be highest in authority. In fact, the more junior members are often more accessible and frequently easier to relate to. The person you choose to coordinate your questions and provide feedback about your progress should be someone who is available, compassionate, and easy to deal with. If he can't answer your questions or give you the information you want, he will communicate with a senior member of the team. The attending staff physician has ultimate responsibility and will undoubtedly spend some time with you to help you understand the consultants' findings, the treatment plan, and your future outlook. But for day-to-day answers and for a rapid conduit to the top, a compassionate junior team member is a valuable friend.

Many answers to your daily questions, such as consultation results, test results, medication or diet changes, queries about your progress or anticipated discharge, will be answered during daily rounds. You should make a list of all of those questions, and have it handy when the doctors arrive. For problems and questions that crop up when the physicians aren't visiting, the physician coordinator with whom you feel most comfortable can be contacted. Ask the nurses to call him. If he can't answer your questions, he can always direct you to the person who can.

Those lowest on the totem pole are generally most accessible to you. In university hospitals most daily health care needs are handled by physicians-in-training and medical students. They are frequently found on your very floor changing dressings, writing orders, examining new patients—in short, disposing of the routine tedious tasks that senior physicians either avoid or are too busy to deal with. These daily duties keep these members of your health care team nearby, within easy reach.

It helps, therefore, to get to know who's who in your health care group. You can find out very simply: (1) ask them; (2) look at name tags. Students' tags don't say "M.D." or "Dr." They generally say "MS1," "MS2," etc. (indicating medical student first year, second year, etc.) The tags of the physicians-in-training will all say "M.D." They may also indicate their training year, or they may merely indicate their specialty (medicine, surgery, pediatrics, psychiatry).

Learn the names of your team members, particularly the one or two with whom you feel most comfortable. Then if you need or want something, you can ask the nurse to call Dr. Jones, rather than "the chubby one who has brown hair and wears glasses."

❧

WHEN TO MAKE SPECIAL REQUESTS
OF THE DOCTOR

In your admission examination the doctor or doctors will ask you what medications you take, whether you have any allergies, and other pertinent questions. If you have any habits, needs, or special requests, the doctor's first visit is a good time to ask. Perhaps you would like a favorite laxative, a particular low-salt diet, a glass of milk at bedtime, a sleeping pill, or even a shot of whiskey before dinner. (Yes, that is often permitted and sometimes even encouraged.) Explain your requests to your examining physician. If they are reasonable and don't interfere with your treatment plan or with hospital policy, he should try to accommodate you.

❧

HOW TO MINIMIZE MISTAKES

Don't be afraid to ask questions; they are one of your major tools in the hospital setting. Not only do you have the right to; you owe it to yourself to do so. Patients are frequently timid, afraid to inquire. Too often they are caught off guard by unexpected arrivals of consultants, unplanned trips to the X-ray department, or unanticipated special studies. They dutifully take whatever medications they are given and eat whatever foods they are served, even if they suspect that something is amiss: and think (but may be afraid to ask) "This isn't my usual low-salt diet," or "I don't recognize these pills." If you know, in no uncertain terms, what your physicians want you to eat and what medicines you should be taking, then speak out if something strikes you as unusual or unexpected. On rare occasion a patient may even find himself heading to the operating room for someone else's procedure. Usually this kind of error is uncovered in the various checks along the way, or the patient is wise enough to scream loudly, "You've got the wrong person!" This sort of Mack Sennett scenario is no fairy tale. It has happened. None of the personnel picked up the error and the patient, certain that the doctors and the hospital knew best, never spoke up. Perhaps the doctor told you in the morning that you would need strict bed rest for five more days. Two hours later the transport crew comes to move you to physical therapy. Don't go until you've ironed out this discrepancy. Ask your doctor. Perhaps they've come for the wrong patient.

A medical student comes into your room with a pint of blood and prepares to give you a transfusion. You don't know this young man. No one told you that you needed a transfusion. You are confused. Don't accept the transfusion without conferring with a senior member of your medical team. The blood may not be for you. Another common error is a patient unwittingly eating a breakfast that should have been withheld, resulting in the cancellation of an operation or special X-ray studies. More serious, we have learned of occasions when patients, mistakenly fed shortly before surgery—an error which nobody noticed—vomited and choked to death during anesthesia. Why? The nurses made a mistake. Had those patients questioned their physicians the night before, they could have recognized the errors themselves.

Asking questions, being sure that you know what's about to happen before it does, becoming involved in your health care program is important for two reasons: the patient who knows what's coming is less anxious and better able to deal with annoying, uncomfortable, unfamiliar tests and procedures; and even more importantly, the informed patient can intervene to help eliminate mistakes. Here are some questions you should ask:

ON ADMISSION:

· What do you think is wrong with me? (He may not know. "That's what you're here to find out," he may say.) But he *can* share his thoughts and plans.)

· What tests will I have and when? Is there any special preparation for any of these tests (for example, fasting)?

· What medications are you ordering? What are they for? What do they look like? How often will I be given them?

• Will I see the anesthesiologist before the operation? What preparations are required before surgery?

AS TIME PASSES:

• What are the test results?

• What did the various consultants think?

• Any changes in medications?

• Any changes in diet?

• How long a recovery period is anticipated?

It may help to write down these or any others that you think of. Lapses of memory can easily occur during hasty afternoon physician rounds. If you exclaim "Hold it a moment! I've got a written list of questions," it may take them by surprise, but they'll answer willingly, and you'll feel more satisfied and in greater control.

Once you are privy to the test and treatment plan, use the information as a source of comfort—the known is always less frightening than the unknown—and as a red flag for potential nursing errors. That doesn't mean that you should anticipate an error or view every recommendation with suspicion. It does mean that an unexpected or unfamiliar shot, procedure, diet, transfusion, or pill should be questioned: What is it? Who ordered it? And if you get an unsatisfactory answer, you should have the order corroborated.

WHEN AND HOW TO CHANGE DOCTORS

It isn't easy to change doctors in midstream. It can be an emotionally disruptive experience. But if you are unhappy with your care, if you are dissatisfied with the anwers to your questions, if your progress is poor and your physicians can't help you understand why, you may be a candidate for a fresh approach. You may want another opinion, a consultation with a specialist, or a transfer to someone else's care.

Friends and relatives are valuable allies in stressful situations like these. They may be more mobile, more rational, and better able to communicate with your doctor than you are. If your communications with the doctors have reached an impasse, ask your closest friend or a relative or a staff social worker to help. Perhaps one of them will be able to bridge the gap between you and your doctor. If you are still worlds apart, request a special visit from your physician when your friend or relative can be with you to offer support. Explain your dissatisfaction: Does he want to operate, but you aren't sure he should and would like another opinion? Are you taking much longer than you expected to get back on your feet? After scores of studies and tests are you no closer to an answer than you were when you entered the hospital?

When your doctor buzzes in and out do you feel as though you are not getting adequate attention? A frank face-to-face discussion is always best. We can't tell you what your doctor's reaction will be. That depends on what you say, how you say it, and what type of person he is. He may be able to allay your concerns and give you a clearer understanding of your problems. He may offer to transfer you to someone else's care or to bring in a consultant. He may rant and rave and go storming out of the room. If he does that, you'd be well advised to change doctors at once, but you probably shouldn't rely on him for a recommendation. In strained and, fortunately, unusual circumstances like these, you must find a new physician yourself. The chief of the department in the hospital is a good choice. Or you may get recommendations from friends, relatives, your personal physician (if your run-in was with a consultant or a surgeon to whom he referred you), or from your local medical society.

11

Understanding Procedures and Equipment: A Good Way to Lessen Your Anxiety

Fifty years ago the hospital laboratory was an extremely primitive place by today's standards. The most significant tools were the microscope and the bacteriologic plate. Body fluids, such as sputum, urine, and blood, were stained with dyes and examined microscopically. There were chemical tests to evaluate gastric (stomach) secretions for acid content, but no analytic studies of blood. There were no respiratory assistive devices, transfusions, or intravenous fluids. Leeches and maggots were still part of the hospital's pharmacy. X-rays had just become commercially available.

With our ever-expanding technology we are now able to see inside the head or body without surgery; analyze blood for its most minute chemical components; follow the moment-to-moment changes in blood oxygen content; and visually and continuously observe the heart rate, blood pressure, and electrocardiogram.

The purpose of this chapter is to describe some of the new and the old technology, so that when you are faced with it you will be less frightened and less intimidated by it. The physicians, technicians, and nurses with whom you come in contact are genuinely trying to help you, not hurt you. Cooperation, relaxation, and understanding can contribute a great deal to your comfort during any special procedures or testing.

❦

LABORATORY STUDIES AND PROCEDURES

Blood Tests

Just about every patient admitted to the hospital will have a complete blood count (CBC), serology (a test for syphilis), and a urinalysis. In most states this is required by law as a minimum base line. Recently some states have legislated that every hospitalized female above eighteen must be offered a Pap smear (cellular smear from the cervix to detect cancer). You, as the patient, have a right to refuse, but the test must be offered.

The CBC and serology are simple blood tests performed in every hospital lab. Either you will go to the lab as part of preadmission testing or the lab technician, nurse, medical student, or other physician will come to your bedside to withdraw a blood sample from a vein.

A needle prick is slightly painful. If you hold still, the discomfort should be brief. Getting a needle in a patient's vein is not always easy, and it may take more than one puncture to accomplish the task. If a blood sample cannot be obtained by the third try, we would suggest that you acknowledge your discomfort and the blood drawer's frustration and request a brief respite. Besides bringing some relief, another more experienced person may take over.

Blood samples will most likely be drawn in the morning before breakfast, since many tests require fasting for greatest accuracy. Therefore, during your first days in the hospital, before you eat breakfast, check with the nurse to be sure that blood tests haven't been ordered. Diabetes, anemias, infections, gout, electrolyte disturbances, and many other disorders necessitate almost daily blood testing in order to guide the physician's management of your illness.

Urinalysis

Urine samples are usually no problem; you void in a container. There are, however, other types of urine tests necessitating a clean-catch specimen, a catheterized sample, or a twenty-four-hour collection. The clean-catch involves a careful cleansing of the genital area, followed by a partial emptying of the bladder, then voiding the first portion of the (residual) urine into a sterile container. The catheterized sample is prepared in a similar manner except that the urine is obtained by placing a tube into the bladder. A twenty-four-hour urine sample is a timed collection of every drop excreted. If you are asked to provide a twenty-four-hour collection, be sure that you understand the directions fully. Starting and stopping times, for example, are very important.

Miscellaneous Laboratory Studies

Other lab studies may be more complex, requiring the assistance of a physician or special expert. Consider, for example, a bone-marrow study that may be needed to evaluate certain blood abnormalities. It is usually the pathologist or hematologist who obtains a bone-marrow sample. The skin and underlying tissues are numbed with a local anesthetic. A special needle is then introduced into an area of spongy bone, either the breastbone (sternum) or the posterior pelvis (iliac crest). This test is extremely important in most forms of anemia or other blood diseases. The area from which the bone-marrow sample was obtained may feel bruised for several weeks after you've left the hospital, but the valuable, and perhaps lifesaving, information obtained from such a test is well worth the transitory discomfort. You may refuse this or any test, but doing so may make it impossible for your physician to diagnose or treat the condition about which you are both concerned.

Spinal Tap

Sometimes it is necessary to examine the spinal fluid, especially in stroke patients, individuals suspected of having meningitis, an numerous other neurologic disorders. This procedure is performed by a physician, frequently a neurologist or neuro-surgeon. The skin over the lower back (lumbar spine) is thoroughly cleansed. A local anesthetic is injected into the skin and underlying tissues. As soon as the area is numb, a long very thin needle is delicately inserted into the spinal canal. A small amount of spinal fluid is allowed to flow into three separate vials and is then sent to the lab for analysis.

The spinal tap is the same procedure used in spinal anesthesia, saddle blocks (anesthesia used during obstetrical delivery), and myelograms (injection of a substance in order to X-ray the spinal canal). Although slightly uncomfortable, it is *not* a painful experi-ence, and an understanding of the procedure should help you banish any undue anxiety. The tap is performed with the patient either sitting in a chair or lying in bed on one side with the legs tucked up. As long as you remain still and relax, it does not hurt. Following the tap, lying flat in bed for four to six hours will usually prevent a headache.

Bacteriology

Bacteriologic examinations are usually done on body or tissue fluids to determine the organism that is responsible for an infec-tion. A sample of urine, blood, pus, sputum, spinal fluid, stool, or almost any other material is smeared onto a medium that encour-ages the growth of bacteria. The resultant bacterial colonies are then bombarded with a large variety of antibiotics so that your physician will know which antibiotic will be most effective in resolving your infection.

Cytology and Histology

Cytology and histology are technologic tools of the patholo-gist. Cells or tissues are removed from the body, applied to a microscopic slide, stained with a variety of dyes, and interpreted diagnostically. Whether a biopsied mass is malignant or benign is urgent information needed by the surgeon to guide the extent of surgery. The pathologist, a vital contributor to the health care team, has the expertise to make this decision.

Radiology and Nuclear Medicine

In this atomic age, the term "radiation" has gotten a great deal of bad press. Without today's medically safe forms of radiation, the medical profession would be severely handicapped. I can't imagine diagnosing an intestinal lesion without the aid of X-ray studies. Some of the newer radiologic techniques not only aid in localizing tumors but can also help in distinguishing between malignant and benign tumors. The CAT scanner enables us to appreciate structural distortions inside the head or body without surgery. And a wide variety of radioactive isotopes can pinpoint diseased organs with amazing accuracy.

It is not necessary to explore with you every test and study in these specialties. We are trying to convey a sufficient understanding of these special areas so that you can intelligently interact with your physician, ask appropriate questions, and consider the risks of medical intervention with less anxiety.

You're familiar with the simple chest X-ray. You stand next to the film and the picture is snapped. Then the radiologist interprets the organ shadows and densities, suggesting diagnostic possibilities to your physician.

Not all organs can be identified so easily. The intestinal tract must first be outlined with barium, swallowed (upper GI series), or instilled rectally (barium enema). The kidneys are visualized by an intravenous dye which concentrates in that organ (IVP). Dye in capsule form is swallowed, metabolized, and excreted into the gallbladder, clarifying any disease in that structure (gallbladder series).

Some organs or parts of organs can only be visualized indirectly by filling their blood vessels with dye. The aorta, blood vessels of the heart, pancreas, or brain require this *angiographic* approach. As mentioned in Chapter 2, not all hospitals perform these sophisticated angiographic studies, and some hospitals that do, shouldn't.

The recent advent of the CAT scanner may revise the need for the more complex angiographic studies. Computerized axial tomography (CAT) allows the radiologist to view regions of the brain or body without injecting dyes. In brief, the patient lies on an X-ray table while the machine takes many pictures that are read and interpreted by a computer. At present the CAT scanner is most effective in detecting tumors, intracranial hemorrhages, or masses. Knowledge regarding other organs is still infantile and needs growth and maturation before the medical profession can rely on this space-age diagnostic tool.

Another dimension in diagnosis is provided by nuclear medicine. The injection of certain radioactive chemical substances expands our ability to observe the structure and function of internal organs that previously could only be guessed at or measured indirectly with less accuracy.

Radioactive scanning has been made possible by expanding on the Geiger counter, a device which measures radioactivity. Radioactivity-tagged chemicals injected intravenously are selectively broken down or concentrated in specific organs. You then lie or sit in front of a scanning machine that counts the radioactive particles.

The radioactivity is of such short duration or low level to preclude any harm to you. The information gathered by this approach outweighs any minute risk except during pregnancy, when the vulnerable fetus may be affected. In pregnant women, these procedures should be avoided except under the most extraordinary circumstances.

A specific type of radioisotope scanning is used to evaluate the thyroid gland. Although there are certain chemical tests that can measure thyroid function, none can delineate the shape of the gland, pick out spots where it is under- or overactive, or search for faraway thyroid cancer metastases the way radioactive iodine scanning can. In some cases, higher dosages of this material are even used therapeutically to destroy malfunctioning thyroid tissue, obviating the need for surgery.

TECHNIQUES AND EQUIPMENT

Blood Transfusion

Blood banks are no longer a mystery to the general public. You've been exposed to Red Cross campaigns and community drives for blood donors. Receiving blood may be lifesaving, but carries a small risk of hepatitis (viral infection involving the liver), serum sickness, or transfusion reactions. In order to prevent or avoid this risk, patients undergoing elective surgery might ask their physicians about *autologous* blood transfusions.

If you know that you need an operation that has been planned for up to three weeks in the future, it may be possible for you to be your own blood donor. As many as three units of whole blood can be withdrawn and stored in anticipation of your operation. In the meantime your body will actively replenish the loss prior to the surgery.

Respiratory Assistive Devices

There is probably nothing more frightening to a parent than a gasping child in respiratory distress. This emergency situation commonly requires dramatic medical intervention. The child must be brought to a hospital where a tracheostomy, or artificial airway, can be created immediately. The team of experts includes a respiratory specialist who quickly hooks up a respirator. The child's breathing becomes less labored and the pale cheeks become pink.

Your grandfather, who used to work in the coal mines, is brought to the hospital because his breathing is rapid and shallow, and his usually ruddy complexion has a dusky overcast. He has chronic obstructive lung disease, and he can't get rid of carbon dioxide or get enough oxygen. A tube is placed into his trachea (endotracheal tube), and a breathing machine takes over the bellows function of his diseased lungs.

The variety of respirators to assist or take over the breathing function has proliferated during the last several years. The Karen Ann Quinlan case in New Jersey has made the public aware of how these devices cannot only save lives but also prolong lives that may not be salvageable.

Nowhere in the hospital are respirators more obvious than in the intensive care units. The rhythmic clicks and hums fill the room with a droning background noise. But as a patient you will most likely be exposed to the simpler devices that help to supply oxygen either by mask or nasal cannula (tube) or that encourage deeper respirations to expand lungs and promote expulsion of respiratory secretions. This latter equipment includes the IPPB (intermittent positive pressure breathing) apparatus, a machine which actively inflates the lungs during inspiration, and a spirometer, a gadget which enables the physician to observe how effectively the patient is expelling air from the lungs. Many physicians prescribe these measures pre- and postoperatively to prevent pulmonary complications. A respiratory therapist should instruct you in the use of this equipment.

Tubes

The body is like a chemical factory producing and nourishing tissue cells continuously and expelling waste products in the process. When one or more of these chemical systems break down or become damaged, a tube may be needed to drain waste, to overcome an obstruction, to prevent blockage, to provide nutrition, or to measure by-products.

For example: many women will temporarily have catheters in their bladders following routine pelvic surgery like hysterectomies; after an appendectomy or other abdominal operation, you may, for a day or two, require a nasogastric tube (running through your nose into your stomach) to keep your bowel at rest; if for any reason you won't be able to eat for a day or two, intravenous fluids will probably be provided; if you've had any kind of chest surgery, you'll need chest tubes for several days to properly keep your lungs inflated.

Devices like these are not extraordinary; they are relatively routine. Therefore, if you find yourself connected in some unnatural way to the outside world, it doesn't necessarily mean there is a problem. Patients are often surprised and confused by these pieces of strange equipment. We recently heard a patient comment, "They took two of those tubes out of me yesterday. Either I'm getting better or they've given up hope."

We will talk more about these special procedures, equipment, and devices in Chapter 14.

12

Labor and Delivery: Why Alternative Methods of Childbirth Necessitate a More Knowledgeable Consumer

Hospitals, refuges for sick people, seem incongruous places for normal, healthy young women about to give birth. Little wonder that scores of women are turning their backs on hospitals and are electing to have their babies at home. They reject the depersonalized institutions and opt for the warmth and family involvement that home deliveries offer. Still other women, who haven't rejected hospitals entirely, will accept them on their own terms. "Natural childbirth," as natural as the hospital can make it, is the path they select.

HOME VERSUS HOSPITAL—THE DETERMINING CRITERIA

Originally, babies were born at home out of need. There was no other choice. In most non-Western societies, that still holds true.

As hospitals proliferated in this country, more and more deliveries moved from the woman's own bed to the hard table in delivery suites. Today many obstetricians and a rapidly expanding corps of nurse-midwives have returned deliveries to the home. Women want this; professionals comply.

The philosophy is unimpeachable. Bringing the baby into the world in its own home, away from crowded nurseries, shielded from the noises and lights of the frenetic hospital, is a most appealing concept. Hospitals are cold, impersonal places: the joy of childbirth is meant to be shared with loved ones rather than with strangers.

As humanitarians, we agree fully with the principles that underlie the move toward home deliveries. As physicians, however, we cannot, in good conscience, endorse the practice.

In most cases (90 to 95 percent) childbirth proceeds smoothly for both mother and newborn. For these uncomplicated events the hospital is, indeed, superfluous. In fact, most deliveries don't even require the services of an attending physician or nurse. If we could always predict accurately which deliveries would be perfectly normal and which might run into trouble, home deliveries would pose no problem. The normal 90 to 95 percent could safely be delivered at home, the others could take place in the hospital. Unfortunately, not all potential hazards can be detected or predicted beforehand. Without any prior warning, acute emergencies do crop up that without the immediate availability of full hospital resources can lead to catastrophic injuries.

Everyone knows that mothers and babies used to die or be injured in childbirth far more often in pioneer days than they are today. Some of those injuries, such as postpartum infections, can be prevented today, even at home, with proper sterilization methods, and the use of antibiotics later if the need arises. But many of those deaths and injuries can be averted only if the child is born in the hospital.

A few years ago one of us worked in a small California hospital. An upsurge of home deliveries, primarily assisted by two obstetricians, was the latest practice—this was in 1970, long before the practice caught on in the rest of the country. I personally saw seven major delivery disasters rushed to our emergency department. In one case the mother died from a sudden, massive, unexpected hemmorrhage. In three cases the babies died because of complications of delivery. In three others the babies and mothers survived, but the children were severely and permanently brain damaged. The tragedy was that all of these deaths and injuries could have been prevented if childbirth had taken place in the hospital.

All physicians have encountered unexpected emergencies during delivery: the baby's umbilical cord may prolapse (fall out before the baby is born), the blood supply to the infant is cut off; unpredictable impediments to fetal circulation can arise while the baby is still inside the mother (these can kill the child or destroy its vulnerable brain); the baby's head or shoulders can get stuck on the way out; severe maternal hemorrhaging can occur. In the hospital there are resources and facilities to handle these emergencies. Sophisticated fetal monitoring equipment to keep constant tabs on the baby's heart rate is available for use as necessary. Emergency Cesarean section can quickly remove a baby in trouble. Special forceps, judiciously applied and manipulated by skilled personnel, can be used to extract (gently) a baby that is stuck. Blood transfusions are instantly available to combat shock and save the life of a bleeding mother. Injuries both to mother and child can occur in the hospital too, but hospital facilities and personnel reduce the chances of such injuries.

Proponents of home deliveries argue that these occurrences are rare and that prompt transportation to a hospital via ambulance can effectively handle most of these emergencies. There is some validity to those arguments, but the key word is "most." Serious emergencies like these may occur only once in every few hundred deliveries, and a fifteen- or twenty-minute trip to the hospital is often time enough to provide proper intervention. But, as we saw from my emergency department experience, irreversible tragedies can and do occur when babies are born at home.

Although the chances of such catastrophes are relatively small, tempting fate with home deliveries means playing for very high stakes. When complications occur, they are almost invariably catastrophic: the mother may lose her life; the baby may not survive; or worst and most common, the fetal blood flow is partially lost. This results in devastating, lifelong neurological injuries. Tragic children, mentally retarded or crippled by cerebral palsy, can be the price that a mother pays for the comfort of childbirth at home.

The hospital environment, cold and impersonal though it may be, offers indispensable emergency resources. Whenever possible, deliveries should take place in hospitals.

⚜

HOW TO GET THE BEST OF BOTH WORLDS— NEW ALTERNATIVES HOSPITALS ARE NOW OFFERING

Although our medical knowledge assures us that hospitals provide the safest delivery settings, our sentiments lie with those who are fighting for a return to "the good old days" of natural, family-oriented deliveries. The best alternative, we believe, is for hospitals to provide more homelike, less "intervention-inclined" facilities for labor and delivery. They should be ready to provide all of their resources at a moment's notice, but to keep out of the way, as much as possible, until those resources are needed.

Some hospitals, prodded by modern-thinking obstetricians, have begun to offer this type of delivery environment. At the furthest (and probably most ideal) extreme, some are providing special delivery rooms that simulate home bedrooms. They permit family members, in most cases fathers, to attend the delivery, and they offer many comforts of home for the mother and her new baby.

A few hospitals are experimenting with the appealing system devised by Dr. Leboyer of France. His philosophy is that birth in the usual hospital setting is severely traumatic to the newborn. The child is viciously extracted from its quiet warm environment and thrust directly into the brightly lit noisy delivery room—its first experience with the outside world. Leboyer, and now a few of his American followers, dim the delivery room lights, eliminate extraneous noises, place the mother in a more natural sitting position, and gently extract the baby. They then immediately place the baby in a warm water bath to simulate its familiar home of the previous nine months. Obstetricians who have adopted this method insist that these newborns smile immediately and seem to be better adjusted children. Proof of these claims is still lacking, and we don't really know what effect this gentle delivery process will have in the long run. But at this point the Leboyer technique is most important for the philosophy it sets forth. It is an attempt to remove the confusion and depersonalization that surrounds most modern hospital deliveries. It espouses the marvelous concept that birth is not a disease or a pathological process; rather it is a normal, natural event that should be treated with dignity, love, and compassion.

The natural childbirth methods of Lamaze, Bradley, hypnosis, and many others are the ones most familiar to all of you. These systems are now widespread and available in nearly every community in the country. They, too, are a progressive move to return pregnancy and delivery to their proper normal status. The most important features of these methods is that they involve the husband in the delivery process, and they strive to minimize the dependency of the laboring woman on medications for pain control. In a recent book coauthored by one of the authors of this book and his physician wife (R. E. Gots and B. A. Gots, *Caring For Your Unborn Child,* Stein and Day, New York, 1977), they explained the various risks associated with pain-relieving and tranquilizing medications. Many of the more commonly used drugs get into the baby's system and depress him. They can interfere with his ability to take that first critical breath.

We wholeheartedly support the various natural childbirth methods. We believe that the emotional support that the father brings can be invaluable; his participation in the birth process brings him closer to his newborn and returns some of the family quality to delivery; and that the fewer medications the mother needs, the better.

The International Childbirth Education Association (CEA), whose national headquarters is in New York City, has local chapters in all major metropolitan areas and in many many smaller towns. You can find a number listed for this organization in the white pages of the telephone book. The avowed purpose of this international organization is to educate women about childbirth. It promotes research and dialogue and teachings about current practices in childbirth. Their literature is available for free or at nominal charge.

In addition, the CEA, its multiple member organizations, and other non-CEA groups sponsor childbirth education classes for interested women. Some are held in local hospitals, others in schools and community centers. Pregnant women in the last six to eight weeks of their pregnancy take these classes. Natural childbirth— Lamaze, Bradley, and other techniques—is taught, demonstrated, and discussed. Husbands are asked to attend and actually participate in learning the techniques. Films are shown of actual deliveries, and the advantages of nearly drug-free deliveries are heavily emphasized.

Even if you do not know if you are interested in natural childbirth techniques, CEA has valuable information to impart, and you would do well to at least call and speak with someone there, get some literature, or even attend a few of the classes. In some areas CEA organizations are broadening the scope of their classes offered. Some offer classes for educating the prospective parents in the care and feeding of babies and children. Others are finding it important to offer support classes for new parents facing the difficulties of having a baby. Your local CEA chapter or office can help you find out which classes are available.

જ્જ

FINDING A PHYSICIAN WHO SHARES YOUR GOALS IN CHILDBIRTH

Many women have an obstetrician-gynecologist even before they become pregnant. Once pregnant, hopefully you will find your doctor a sympathetic, understanding physician. However, as you begin to learn more about pregnancy and childbirth, you may find that you and your doctor may have an unbridgeable chasm between you. He may pooh-pooh your concerns about drugs during pregnancy or delivery, or he may find absurd your interest in natural childbirth techniques or in Leboyer.

Don't feel committed to a particular doctor if you are so widely separated on such vital issues. You may ask friends for a reference to another physician with whom you might find you have more in common philosophically. Another very important referral service is the CEA itself. This organization and its member chapters keep a listing of those obstetricians who are sympathetic to the concepts espoused by the CEA organizations. Other sources include the local hospital, and the nearest university medical center. Another good way to find a sympathetic obstetrician is by attending some childbirth education classes in your area: here you can get the advice of both the instructor and, perhaps, other women who have had firsthand experiences.

If you don't have a physician when you become pregnant, the same areas of investigation are open to you. Search carefully—for you are choosing the physician who is going to be responsible for your welfare and that of your child during this most crucial period of both your lives. His or her expertise will, to a great extent, determine the safety of your child's passage into this world.

The quality of an obstetrician is more easily judged by the consumer than nearly any other type of medical or surgical specialist. For the most part, obstetrical practice is taking care of healthy women going through a natural process. You most need a physician's care when something goes awry during pregnancy or when the progress of labor and delivery is suddenly interrupted by a problem. What is needed then, is a vigilant, caring doctor who is alert to you and sympathetic to your concerns and problems. If a particular individual is unwilling to answer your questions, seems abrupt when you inquire about drugs, diet, or alternative labor and delivery techniques, or seems not to listen to your symptoms or brushes them aside despite your obvious concern, then he is not the physician for you.

After you have pursued these various courses of investigation we have suggested and have several possible names, you should then seek out and speak with a few patients of these physicians if that is possible. Finally, meet with the doctors yourself. Again, don't feel obligated to the physician you had during your routine pelvic exams and Pap smears. Pregnancy intimately involves you, your unborn child, and your physician. The physician you choose should display an interest in you and your questions and a vigilance over your progress and symptoms, for this is a positive indication of both sensitivity and clinical competency.

❦

DRUGS FOR LABOR AND DELIVERY—HOW TO AVOID THE QUIET TRAP AND STILL PROTECT YOUR BABY

Although you may fervently decide beforehand that you will give birth with no external aids, you may find that you need some relief once labor is in full force. If so, you should accept the medications you need without guilt or shame. Everybody's needs are different. Moreover, if the right drugs are provided in as small dosages as possible, the risk to your baby can be minimized. For those of you who will get some pain relievers (most of you, to be sure), we will briefly discuss obstetrical anesthetics so that you will know which agents are safest.

First of all, take some initiative. Have a discussion with your obstetrician before your due date. Let him know that if you want pain relief you would like to share in the decision of what and when, otherwise you may get a "routine" pain shot even if you don't need it.

No drugs are completely safe; all can depress the baby to some extent. The most potent depressants are narcotics like morphine and Demerol, followed by commonly used tranquilizers like Valium and barbiturates. Local anesthetics that are given, such as spinal, epidural, caudal, and saddle blocks, are relatively safe if the baby is carefully monitored. Small doses of nitrous oxide (laughing gas), the anesthetic that you commonly breathe in dentists' offices, is also fairly safe if administered judiciously, in small amounts, when absolutely needed.

Labor and delivery can be a difficult experience for the mother and stressful period for the about-to-be-born child. The ideal goal is to make the event as comfortable as possible for the mother, always mindful of the safety of the unborn child. At times this may require some delicate balancing or leaning in the direction of the child. Mother's pain will be short lived, but an over-medicated child may suffer permanent injury and bring anguish to himself and his family for the rest of his life. The rules are simple:

childbirth education classes and natural (no drug) childbirth if possible; pain relief, if necessary, by local anesthetic blocks; a few breaths of nitrous oxide if supplemental relief is needed; narcotics and other depressant medications only as a last resort, to be avoided as much as possible.

❧

SELECTING THE BEST OBSTETRICIAN AND OBSTETRICAL HOSPITAL

For the majority of normal uncomplicated deliveries any hospital will do. However, 5 to 15 percent of deliveries are not completely normal. In a moment of crisis, there is no substitute for experienced, up-to-date specialized obstetrical nursing care.

In many hospitals, the laboring woman won't see a physician right away. In fact, if she is in early labor, she may remain solely in the hands of the nursing staff for many hours. The nurses perform pelvic examinations to determine the degree of cervical dilation and the station of the baby—both are measures of the progress of labor and the nearness to delivery. Nurses time contractions, listen with a stethoscope for the fetal heart sounds, or hook up monitoring equipment that does this automatically. This vigilance is vitally important, for a change in fetal heart rate is an early red flag—a sign of fetal distress.

In an ideal world, constant nurse monitoring, and physician attendance throughout all of labor would offer the best chance of saving mothers and babies in trouble. At the moment, that goal is rarely achievable. Hospitals cannot support one nurse per patient (even if they could, they never know how many women in labor will arrive at a time), and a physician can't possibly sit by his patient's bedside for six to twenty hours. You can only hope to come as close to those ideals as possible. At the very least, you want specialized obstetrical nurses to evaluate you every fifteen or twenty minutes. Your physician should be no more than a half-hour away during early labor and on the spot or down the hall for the last couple of hours.

Well-trained obstetrical nurses can identify problems as they develop, if they watch you closely. It pays to check out the obstetrical service of your hospital before you have to go. If you have two or more choices of hospitals, opt for the one with the best obstetrical service. Talk to your physician, your friends, and the appropriate hospital spokesperson—in this case either the administrator, the public information office, or the director of nursing. Review the labor room protocol. How often do the nurses check each patient? Are all of the nurses specialized in obstetrical care? Do they have an active obstetrical service—two or three babies per day at least? If not, the hospital down the road where ten babies enter the world each day may be better equipped and better staffed to handle the broadest range of obstetrical needs.

When it comes to obstetrical care, choosing the most concerned, sympathetic, conscientious obstetrician will often automatically lead you to the right hospital. The reason is that the obstetrician and his patients are so dependent on competent nursing that a top-notch obstetrician will either avoid the hospital with a mediocre nursing service, or he will personally work with the administration to shore up the weaknesses. When a nurse calls him at 3:00 A.M. and tells him that his patient is only three centimeters dilated—hours away from delivery—he counts on her to be accurate. When she informs him that all is well with the baby, he must be able to trust her judgment. If he can't and he cares about *his* patients, he'll soon be spending twenty-four hours a day every day sitting with his patients in labor.

You'll want to discuss your doctor's delivery routine with him (and other patients of his—an excellent source of information) long before your due date. In fact, that discussion should be an important piece of decision-making data as you select an obstetrician. Does he expect to be away at delivery time? Does he share nighttime delivery duties with one or more associates? If you get positive answers to these questions, you'd be well advised to inquire about and personally meet his colleagues. There is nothing more disconcerting than to find your ideal obstetrician only to confront an unfamiliar, and perhaps less concerned, less competent, individual at the most critical moment of all—when labor is well under way. Other questions about your doctor's delivery routine should include: When does he come to the hospital? (It's all right if he defers to good nursing judgment in the early stages, but you don't want him popping in as your baby's head is halfway out. He should plan to arrive by the time your cervical dilation has reached 6 or 7 centimeters.) How far is he from the hospital? (The closer the better. If he is too far away, he cannot respond promptly to an emergency.)

※

THINGS YOU SHOULD KNOW ABOUT LABOR AND DELIVERY PROCEDURES

Once you are in active labor, you aren't in the best position to organize things. That's why careful prescreening of your doctor and hospital is so important. You should be evaluated every fifteen minutes at least. The most important aspect of that regular exam is listening for the fetal heart sounds or reviewing the monitoring record. Pelvic examinations are done less often. Your doctor should be on his way once your cervix is five or six centimeters dilated. If you see a nurse only every hour, or if your doctor has not been informed of the upcoming delivery—now only one hour away—call out. Confront the nurse and complain. Better yet, if your husband is with you have him do it. At that point he'll be in a much stronger position than you.

It pays to stay informed. Insist on regular progress reports from the nurses and the doctor, once he arrives. A physician friend was recently forced to intervene actively when his wife's obstetrician made a foolish error. She was completely dilated at ten centimeters, but the baby had not quite moved down into the delivery position. The obstetrician decided that delivery was at least an hour away, although he had no real way of knowing, and he moved toward the door to go to a party across the street. Our physician friend literally blocked the door and physically restrained him. It was fortunate, for fifteen minutes later the baby got into trouble and an emergency Cesarean section promptly followed.

If labor is progressing poorly—either your contractions are coming and going, cervical dilation is slow, or the baby is advancing slowly—your doctor must come to examine you personally.

There may be a problem that he will have to diagnose and correct. For example, if you have been in labor for ten hours and your cervix has remained stationary at three centimeters, your doctor must come see you. Insist that he be summoned. If for any reason the nurses resist, have your husband call him.

If your labor is being induced or stimulated with Pitocin, an obstetrician (your doctor or a physician-in-training) must be in the hospital and moments away. Stimulated labors can be complicated: quick physician intervention may be needed. Your safest bet is to refuse any labor-stimulating drugs until you have seen a doctor and are assured that he will be nearby.

Episiotomy

An episiotomy is a minioperation used to facilitate vaginal deliveries. In this procedure the obstetrician makes an incision through the lower part of your vaginal area just as the baby is about to emerge. The standard teaching is that this reduces the trauma to the mother and lessens the likelihood of any injury that the baby's head can create. A few critics of the procedure argue that it is unnatural and potentially harmful. Most obstetricians in this country do use this procedure, and we believe that the data support the value of episiotomy in most women, particularly those giving birth for the first time. After the baby is born the episiotomy incision is sewn up by the obstetrician. The surgical site can be painful for a few days after delivery; but the discomfort soon abates, and the incision generally heals promptly and readily.

Cesarean Section

Very simply, Cesarean section is the operation that extracts the baby from the uterus via an abdominal incision rather than through the usual vaginal delivery route. In some cases women have elective Cesarean sections; they know before they go into labor that the operation is planned. This is true for women who have extremely large babies, for some cases of breech (foot first) fetal presentations, and for some who have had previous deliveries by Cesarean section. However, the old rule "once a Cesarean section always a Cesarean section" is no longer generally accepted by obstetricians. Women with adequate-sized pelvises, who have had one previous Cesarean section operation for an acute problem in labor, can subsequently deliver vaginally.

Other Cesarean sections aren't planned ahead of time but become necessary because troubles arise during labor. If the mother bleeds severely or if the fetus shows signs of distress or failure to move normally down the birth canal, a Cesarean section may be indicated. Some very knowledgeable, highly respected obstetricians have recently expressed alarm over the increasing frequency of this procedure. Moment-to-moment monitoring of fetal heart rate and other vital functions, now available because of advances in equipment and technology, has, in some cases and in some institutions, produced a phenomenal increase in these operations. In some hospitals, as many as 40 percent of all babies are born this way rather than via the natural vaginal route. Critics believe that many obstetricians, although sincerely concerned about the welfare of the fetus, may be overreacting to minor fetal irregularities and may, as a result, be overusing the operation. If your child is truly in jeopardy Cesarean section may be mandatory, but you have the right and responsibility to know why it is being recommended. Before you agree to the procedure, have your obstetrician explain the indications, the risk, the pros and cons.

13

Surgery: Getting Through It With the Least Stress and Speeding Your Recovery

It is natural for people to have some anxiety when facing surgery (so don't feel guilty or ashamed if you do), but there are many ways to lessen your worry. One of the best ways is to express your fears and find some answers to problems that may be troubling you. What we would like to do is to help you understand what to expect, what questions to ask, and how to help speed your safe recovery.

There are two general classifications of surgical procedures: emergency and elective. Emergency procedures are operations that can't wait. Repairs of an acutely ruptured major artery, surgery for internal injuries suffered in an automobile collision, removal of an inflamed appendix are a few of literally thousands of acute surgical conditions. These life-threatening illnesses and injuries don't give you much time to prepare. The one consolation is that their acute nature offers less opportunity for introspection and worry. Often family members are more anxious than the patients.

Elective surgery is a different matter entirely. These are the planned or scheduled operations. Hysterectomies, cholecystectomies (removal of the gallbladder), many cancer operations, prostate surgery, cataract extractions, removal of torn knee cartilage, cosmetic plastic surgery are a few. Since for these procedures you have days or weeks to ruminate, you may face preoperative jitters. But you do have time to prepare yourself physically, intellectually, and to some extent, emotionally for what lies ahead. Let's talk primarily about these elective operations, since they do permit preplanning. We won't begin to catalog them or to give specific advice for every conceivable operation. That would be an entire book of its own. Instead, here are some general principles that you can apply to many elective operations. At the end of the chapter we provide a list of some common operations; for each we have noted the anesthesia techniques used, the approximate length of hospital stay required, and the usual recovery times.

⤜❦⤏

PREHOSPITALIZATION DISCUSSIONS

First, do you need the operation? By now most of you are aware of the publicity about unnecessary surgery. This has caused considerable public overreaction—suspicion, paranoia, certainty that surgeons are "knife happy." To be sure, unnecessary surgery is a real phenomenon, not a myth, but it isn't as rampant or (most important) as Machiavellian as some would have us believe. There are a small number of surgeons who operate recklessly for minimal indications, for personal gain. Usually, though, arguments over whether surgery is necessary or unnecessary arise from honest differences of opinion; often operative indications aren't clear-cut or well defined. One surgeon may sincerely and properly believe that an operation is indicated; another may disagree. Whether or not "unnecessary surgery" is being overplayed, you do owe it to yourself to feel confident that your recommended operation is truly indicated. A commonsense approach is your best guide.

If you have almost imperceptible visual impairment in one eye and an ophthalmologist tells you the first time you see him that you need immediate cataract surgery, don't pack your suitcase for a trip to the hospital. Get another opinion. On the other hand, if you've seen the same ophthalmologist for six years, and he and you have observed your vision deteriorate progressively during that time, his recommendation for cataract surgery may be accepted without question. In the first place, he hardly rushed the procedure; he demonstrated his willingness to wait and see. In addition, you know that your vision in that eye is now very bad. Common sense tells you that you have a problem that needs to be corrected.

Consider another common and often overprescribed operation: hysterectomy. You are thirty-five years old. You complain to your gynecologist that you had one episode of spotting between periods. He briefly examines you and announces, "Your uterus is enlarged, we'd better take it out." Perhaps he is right. But three months earlier he never mentioned any enlargement, and you really haven't had any symptoms except the one minor bout of spotting. In this case a second gynecological opinion makes sense. Why? Because the doctor's recommendation was hasty and because he suggested a hysterectomy as the first approach. As most women know, usually a D and C (dilation and curettage) precedes a hysterectomy. Moreover, you had no inkling that you might need a hysterectomy: not that a layman would necessarily know, but frequently she would have had enough difficulties to give her a clue. Normally, if an elective operation (other than for cancer surgery) is indicated, the news isn't a total shock.

At the other extreme, perhaps you've had excessive uterine bleeding for several years, have undergone three D and Cs, and have experienced continual pain. Your physician has told you for the past three years that your uterus was enlarged and that you have fibroid tumors. Finally, both of you decide that a hysterectomy (removal of the uterus *only*) is in order. You are not surprised by this, and your doctor managed your problem conservatively for a long time: hardly what you would call a "knife happy" surgeon. Common sense tells you that his suggestion is well founded, and you readily agree to the operation.

This "commonsense approach" to elective surgery, therefore, begins with the following questions: (1) Am I surprised that surgery was suggested, or did I have some inkling that an operation might be necessary? (2) Did the doctor try or suggest other means of therapy before recommending surgery? (3) Did the surgeon observe me for a period of time before suggesting surgery, or was this decision made immediately or very hastily?

These general questions are applicable to most potential non-cancerous surgical problems, but they *do not* apply to suspected malignancies. Don't reject a breast biopsy because a surgeon who feels a lump on your first visit wants to operate immediately. Watchful anticipation has no place when cancer is a possibility.

Once you've made a preliminary commitment to go ahead with the planned surgery, the next step is to get as much information about the surgery as possible. Certain phases of that information gathering are known by the term "informed consent," an ever increasingly common consumer word in this new era of public awareness and physician accountability. Very simply, informed consent means receiving sufficient information from your doctor to allow you to participate actively in the decision and let you know what lies ahead. It includes a discussion of alternative forms of therapy, the pros and cons of surgery—what will happen if you don't have the operation, what you can expect if you do, various types of operative techniques if several options exist—and the risks of surgery.

After you have had this discussion and remain convinced that surgery is the proper approach, you should discuss some other specifics with the doctor. What kind of anesthesia will you use? Who will be administering the anesthesia? (This is the time to speak out and raise those important anesthesia issues we discussed in Chapter 2.) How long will you be in the hospital?

YOUR FIRST DAY IN THE HOSPITAL

In general you will be admitted one or two days before your operation. When you see your surgeon or one of the physicians-in-training for an admission examination, you may want to explore what's to come in more detail. You might want to know how long the incision will be and exactly where it will be located. You may want to ask about any tubes, wires, drains, catheters, or other devices that may protrude from various parts of your body after the operation—not because they are frightening devices, but so that you will understand how they can help in your recovery and so you will not be surprised at finding them. Physicians, used to surgical management, often take these for granted. In following their everyday routines they often forget that the patient is a first-time participant. Patients are often shocked to awaken with tubes in their noses draining their stomach contents; catheters in their bladders collecting their urine; drains protruding from incision sites; tubes in their chest draining air, fluid, or blood; intravenous lines; or occasionally tubes in their tracheas connected to a ventilator artificially supporting respiration (this is not part of usual operative procedures, but it may be used following open-heart or any equally serious operations). The patient who is unprepared for these artificial connectors to the outside world may panic, feeling that something must have gone wrong. If you discuss these often routine measures with your physician beforehand, you can eliminate some postoperative alarm. Knowing what will happen, why it is necessary, and that it is just routine is a great anxiety reliever.

Before you enter a teaching hospital you might want to discuss a matter with your surgeon which probably never occurred to you: Who will be operating? Most people naturally assume that their private surgeon will actually perform the surgery. In fact, teaching hospitals teach surgeons-in-training how to operate in the only way possible—by having them perform operations. Often a private surgeon will permit a trainee to operate on his patients, under his close supervision, naturally. The most complicated procedures he will likely do himself. Less hazardous ones, such as hemorrhoid operations, appendectomies, and hernia repairs, are often done by junior members of the operating team.

If you are comfortable with your surgeon and respect his judgment, you should feel comfortable with his operative discretion. No matter who is the primary operator, your physician is responsible for you. He will permit only an appropriately advanced and skillful surgical trainee to operate. Moreover, he will assist closely, making certain that his pupil is as careful as he would be. If you want nobody but your own doctor to be the head surgeon, tell him. Insist that he and he alone do your operation. Yes, you do have that choice. And today, unlike a few years ago, you will rarely get any argument if you insist that your private surgeon do the operation. But you might be surprised to learn that most patients, when given the choice, are quite willing to permit the junior surgeon to operate.

❦

THE PREOPERATIVE VISIT BY THE ANESTHESIOLOGIST

The night before your surgery you will be visited by the anesthesiologist. He or she can usually tell you what time your operation will be. Find out what types of anesthesia are available—spinal, general, local—and what the options are for your particular operation. In some cases—hemorrhoid procedures, lower extremity operations, many othopedic procedures, eye operations—there are choices. You might choose to be awake or asleep, to have sedation with local anesthesia, spinal anesthesia, or general anesthesia. For other procedures, such as major abdominal surgery, there isn't an option; you will probably be put to sleep with general anesthesia. If you have a choice, the same informed-consent questions that you put to your surgeon are applicable here: What are the pros and cons of the various methods? Which is most advisable? Which is most customary? Which is most dangerous? Most likely you won't be able to eat on the morning of your operation. To be sure, ask the anesthesiologist. Then, if you are mistakenly given breakfast the next day, don't eat it!

Questions the Anesthesiologist Should Ask You

Be sure the anesthesiologist asks you the following relevant questions: (1) Any allergies? (This is very important since many drugs are part of anesthesia management, and the anesthesiologist must be alerted if potential offenders are to be avoided.) (2) Any previous adverse anesthesia experiences? (This, too, is a critical question. For example, approximately 5 percent of normal people react abnormally to the commonly employed drug succinylcholine. This drug is used to paralyze the patient to facilitate artificial respiration. Those who react adversely take an inordinately long time to overcome the drug affect. They remain paralyzed and unable to breathe on their own for an hour or so after the operation is over. The problem is readily managed by mechanical ventilation, but forewarned is forearmed. You can imagine how helpful it would be for the anesthesiologist to be able to anticipate this problem. If you remember or were ever told that you took a long time to come out of an earlier anesthesia, be certain that you inform the anesthesiologist. Perhaps after your last operation the surgeon or anesthesiologist casually mentioned that they had trouble passing the tube into your trachea. That is a critical bit of information to share with the new anesthesiologist.) (3) Have you had any recent operations using general anesthesia? (Certain anesthetic agents can be dangerous if they are repeated after a brief interval of a month or two. If the anesthesiologist knows that you had a general anesthesic one month earlier, he may choose to use a different one this time.) (4) Have you ever had any unexplained fevers following a previous general anesthetic? (Think hard. Some anesthetics may produce a mild reaction the first time, which may be followed by much more serious reactions with subsequent use.)

On the night before your operation you may, quite naturally, feel somewhat apprehensive. Generally your doctor will have ordered a sedative or sleeping medication for you to help soothe you, relieve your anxiety, and help you get a comfortable night's rest. The medication may or may not be given automatically. In other words, the order may be available, but you may have to request it. We would advise you to do so. Even if you feel calm and in control, you will probably have some unconscious tensions that should be relieved.

THE SURGICAL "PREP"

Surgical "prep" is the term used by hospital insiders to describe the physical preparations that you will undergo prior to surgery. Depending on the type of surgery, preps may include: not eating solid food for several days, taking antibiotics if bowel surgery is planned, cleansing and shaving the surgical site, giving you an enema or a laxative to clean out your gastrointestinal tract prior to certain operations, placing a catheter in your bladder in order to irrigate it with cleansing solutions prior to some urological surgery, placing drops in your eyes for a day or two prior to some eye operations.

Occasionally patients who are unprepared for these "preps" may experience some anxiety when faced with an aide or a nurse, razor in hand, ready to shave strategic areas. Understanding what they are all about and that surgical preps are commonplace can help relieve your tensions.

A friend recently became nearly hysterical and summarily dismissed an aide who came to shave her for surgery. The reason: the operation was a mastectomy, but the attendant began shaving her thigh, an area far removed and, as far as she could see, unrelated to the operation. Her immediate thoughts—quite reasonable in view of her lack of preinformation—were that they had either found the wrong patient or that her cancer had spread to her groin, a fact that her doctor hadn't mentioned. Actually the reason for the thigh shaving was quite straightforward. Radical mastectomies sometimes require skin grafting for proper closure of the wound. The thigh is the preferred donor site for the graft, and shaving her thigh was designed to prepare her should she require skin grafting.

The lesson from this and other stories is that preoperative preparations, which may seem unusual to you, the patient, are often required. It will certainly help if you discuss preps with your surgeon beforehand. Knowing exactly what to expect is a remarkable tonic for preoperative jitters that unexpected happenings may otherwise bring.

THE DAY OF SURGERY

Give all valuables to a friend or relative for safekeeping. Everybody knows when you'll be away. Operative schedules are widely available. What better time for any hospital employees who dabble in burglary to raid your bedside drawer. One of our wives, a physician herself, trustingly left a watch in her drawer. When she returned from a one-hour operation, it was gone.

No artifical eyelashes, false teeth, or other removable items are permitted in the operating room. They are hazardous. At the beginning of anesthesia, when the tube is passed down the trachea, patients have choked on broken false teeth that migrated downward into the breathing passages. On the morning of surgery, safety must take precedence over vanity.

An hour or so before your procedure you will usually be given some preoperative medications. These are designed to reduce your anxiety and make the early phases of surgical preparation go more smoothly.

WHAT TO EXPECT IMMEDIATELY FOLLOWING SURGERY

Unless your operation was very minor, using only local anesthesia or mild sedatives, your immediate postoperative respite will be in the recovery room. There patients are lined up one next to the other so that they can be carefully watched by the usually abundant nursing and anesthesia staff. You remain in the recovery room until you are completely awake and your vital signs are stable or until the spinal anesthetic has worn off (if you had a spinal). You can rest assured that the recovery room is where you will get the best supervision and your return to your room signals the fact that all is well. On the evening following your operation your main desire will probably be for rest. Pain-relieving medication, perhaps a light meal, and early sleep will be the program. You should probably plan to minimize visits from friends and relatives that evening.

❦

SELF-HELP FOR POSTSURGICAL DISCOMFORT

As you might expect, there are certain annoyances and discomforts that follow surgery. Fortunately we are now able to control these quite well with simple supportive measures and a vast array of modern medications.

Your doctor will routinely order a variety of drugs to combat most of your postoperative complaints. It is important for you to realize that your doctor's postsurgical orders may not be tailor-made for your very individual needs. As you encounter any discomfort that you would like to control or eliminate, you can help yourself by apprising your doctor or nurse of your difficulties. Don't lie back uncomfortable but close-mouthed thinking that your doctor has prescribed the best or only regimen that can help you. Surgeons each have their own standard routines for managing their just-operated-upon patients. They use medications with which they are most familiar and which, through experience, they have found to be best in most cases. Similarly, the medication dosages and the frequency with which they can be administered are part of the surgeon's standard system. But patients are not all the same. They may respond differently to various medications. Five milligrams of morphine every four hours may provide excellent pain relief for one patient. Another person may need ten milligrams every three hours. Some individuals may find that a certain pain medication causes nausea, but that a substitute is well tolerated. One person may sleep soundly on the night following surgery with no sleeping medication at all. Another patient may require twice the "usual" dosage. What this means for you is that if you find that the pain medication, nausea reliever, sleeping aid, or laxative that your doctor prescribes isn't doing the job, let him know. There are so many alternative medications and dosages available that he should be able to choose one that helps you the most. Or, if you notice that you react poorly to a drug—certain pain relievers can cause nausea, for example—tell your nurse to inform your physician or let him know yourself. He will always be willing to switch to another one. Thus, your postoperative comfort is important, and you are the one who knows best whether you are getting adequate relief. Your doctor needs your help in order to design a drug regimen to fit your personal needs.

We have alluded to a few of the postoperative problems that you may face. Let's consider some of these individually.

Pain

Of course some pain inevitably follows all operations. But the many potent narcotics now available have brought immeasurable relief to the postoperative period. Most can be administered every three or four hours—at first by injection, and after several days, when the pain begins to wane, by mouth. Don't hesitate to request the pain shot that your doctor orders. It may not abolish your pain entirely, but it should take the edge off substantially. If it doesn't, find out why. Can the dosage be increased? Can you get the shots more often? Might another choice be better? Some individuals are inherently more stoic than others; they either don't feel much pain or they don't let it bother them. Other people are more troubled by the pain of an operation, and they may require some sedation along with the pain shot. Generally the combination of a sedative and a narcotic brings substantial relief to even the most sensitive patient.

Various activities aggravate postoperative pain. To some extent these painful maneuvers can be minimized, especially early on; but (as we will see in the next section) they cannot be avoided indefinitely, for movement and exercise encourage speedy recovery. Thus, if you've just had a knee operation, you'll be most comfortable if you keep your leg immobile. When you try to shift around or sit up, you jostle the surgical site and your pain increases. As exercise becomes a necessary part of your recovery program, you learn to ask for your pain shot a half hour or so before your planned trip to the bedside chair (to give it time to achieve its maximal effect). Similarly, if you've had chest surgery, it hurts most to cough and take deep breaths, but coughing and deep-breathing exercises are important. Again you learn to time the pain shot prior to carrying out those activities that are the most painful. A trick that seasoned surgical nurses and physicians learn is that padding and splinting an incisional site can be very helpful. You simply take a pillow and press it against the operative area, as though you were hugging a teddy bear against yourself. This keeps the incision from shaking about and reduces the pain when you get out of bed, walk around, cough, or practice deep-breathing exercises.

Many of the narcotic medications can cause nausea and vomiting. If you notice that you become sick to your stomach after receiving a pain shot, tell the nurse. Often a change of drugs will eliminate the problem since patients frequently tolerate some but not others. If they all bring on the same unpleasant effect, your doctor can order an antinausea medication to be given with the narcotic. That should eliminate this bothersome side affect.

Nausea and Vomiting

Nausea and vomiting are occasional, usually temporary, aftermaths of surgery. General anesthesia may, at times, produce transient stomach upsets. Other causes may be related to the operation itself—if it is an abdominal procedure, for example—reactions to certain medications, or to a food intolerance. Usually the problem is mild and short lived. Eating smaller meals, blander foods, or easy-to-digest foods, such as jello, soups, toast, ice cream, may help. Other self-help remedies include drinking warm tea, ginger ale, or for some people, chewing some ice chips. Many of our patients report that cola beverages are helpful, and for some they might be. Which of these methods may be best for you is hard to predict since patients react differently; but all are worth a try, and you will probably find a regimen that brings relief.

In some cases a specific cause can be found and eliminated. This is particularly true when a drug is the offender. If you find that after receiving your pain shot you become nauseated, tell your doctor and ask him to switch to another medication.

Finally, many drugs are now available for sufferers of nausea and vomiting that can effectively control the symptoms. Your doctor may or may not order these routinely, but if you need one, don't hesitate to ask.

Appetite—Getting Back to Eating

Even those who don't develop actual nausea and vomiting postoperatively may not feel like eating for a few days. A surgical experience seems to dampen the appetite. There are several good ways to get back on the track.

Some physicians begin their patients with jello—a favorite flavor. It is easy to tolerate and cool going down. Most patients accept this very well. Then a little fruit added to the jello is the next step. Once this has been successful for several meals, a gradual move to soft, easy-to-digest foods and then to a regular diet often goes quite smoothly.

Another technique is to begin with just liquids, then mix a small portion of oatmeal, cream of wheat, or another bland cereal with milk. As tolerated, the proportion of cereal is gradually increased until you are eating a regular bowl of cereal. From that point proceed to bland foods—toast, jello, soups, ice cream—then chicken, and finally, full, regular meals.

If you have no dietary restrictions, a favorite delicacy—an ice cream sundae, a milkshake, pizza, or escargots—brought in by a friend or relative may revitalize a temporarily sluggish appetite. Another remedy for that "no-taste-for-food" feeling is a little wine or cocktail before dinner. Many hospitals have wine or hard liquor available. They can be ordered by the physician as a predinner appetite stimulant or a bedtime sedative.

Insomnia

The strange hospital environment combined with postoperative discomfort and daytime dozing can disturb your usual sleep pattern. If you have a home bedtime routine—the evening news, a glass of warm milk, martini—trying (if possible) to approximate this in the hospital can be helpful. In addition you may need some supplementary sleeping aids. Most standard postsurgical orders include a sleeping medication if needed. When the nurse asks you whether you want it, don't hesitate to accept it. Rest is an important aid to prompt recovery.

Urination

This normal bodily function can be disturbed by some anesthetic drugs used for the operation, and certain medications given postoperatively may make voiding difficult.

An even more common cause is postoperative recumbency, which can be a major obstacle to urinating, particularly for men.

A very useful technique that some wise old surgeons employ is to have their male patients practice voiding while lying down (even at home) for few days prior to surgery. Amazingly, simply learning and getting used to this technique can eliminate the postoperative discomfort of a distended bladder.

If you do have difficulty voiding after surgery, the old childhood standbys can work: dipping your fingers in warm water or turning on a nearby faucet are the familiar ones. Having someone help you into the natural standing position (only for men, of course) may enable you to void. Finally, if all else fails, you may need to have a tube passed into your bladder to drain the urine. This is almost pain free for women, but it is somewhat uncomfortable for men. However, by the time you reach that point, the catheter promises such welcome relief that the discomfort is hardly noticed.

Gas Pains, Intestinal Cramps, and Constipation

Anesthetic medications, abdominal operations, postoperative medications, bed rest, and altered eating patterns may temporarily confuse your intestinal tract. The result may be gas pains, some intestinal cramping, and/or constipation.

Gas pains occur when your stomach becomes overfilled due to slowed emptying, or when you swallow too much air. The remedies are quite simple and generally effective. Belching, which can be stimulated by drinking a carbonated beverage, is your easiest and first approach. Antacid medications, such as Maalox, Gelusil, Amphogel, ordered by your physician (at your request), can also bring fast relief.

The medical writer Lawrence Galton reports on the suggestion of a nurse who suffered gas retention after undergoing surgery and came up with the following "telephoning teen-ager" position.

It involves simply lying, stomach down, on a bed, with legs bent at the knees and held up at a comfortable 90-degree angle, and with arms, bent at the elbows, turned toward each other and stretched out ahead and supporting the head held higher than the rest of the body. It is, claims the nurse, a restful position and effective if the gas problem is not too severe—and sometimes also circling the lower legs provides mild abdominal muscle exercise, which aids peristalsis and the expulsion of flatus.*

Abdominal cramps often go hand in hand with postsurgical constipation as the intestine, trying to rid itself of waste materials, contracts and squeezes. In general these problems are quite temporary. They disappear in a few days, after your digestive system readjusts to your new diet and the reduced physical activity that follows surgery. Your physician will probably order a stool softener or mild laxative to control these annoying problems. You may be given this automatically, or you may have to specifically request it. For the most part a mild stool softener, such as mineral oil in orange juice each morning or a natural laxative like prune juice, is the best choice. These help your system get back on a natural track and they combat cramping and constipation. More potent cathartics, such as magnesium citrate, have more intense affects on the intestinal system and they may actually increase cramping. They should only be used if constipation is severe or prolonged.

If cramping is unusually intense, your doctor can prescribe any of a variety of medications that put the bowel to rest. In the postoperative patient these are usually accompanied by a stool softener or mild laxative to combat their constipating actions.

Contrary to common belief, a daily bowel movement is not necessary for good or normal health. Many perfectly normal individuals may move their bowels every other day or only twice weekly. Even if your usual bowel habits dictate a daily evacuation, don't be concerned if that changes temporarily following surgery. Since you will eat very little on the day of surgery and you will be given medications that slow intestinal activity, you may not have a bowel movement for two or three days postoperatively. This is

* From *Save Your Stomach* by Lawrence Galton. © 1977 by Lawrence Galton. Used by permission of Crown Publishers, Inc., New York.

normal, natural, and doesn't signal a problem. As mentioned earlier, mild stool softeners and laxatives can help reinstate a normal bowel pattern. Enemas and more potent laxatives and suppositories can be used if you need urgent relief. But these are only used once the constipation is unduly prolonged or particularly uncomfortable.

Hiccups

Hiccups occasionally bother the postsurgical patient, particularly those who have had abdominal surgery. The cause may be related to stomach distention. If so, the measures described above for managing gas pains may work here. Another trick which we have found very useful is to have patients quickly swallow a large teaspoonful or packet of sugar. This may sound strange, but there have actually been some studies that show why this works (no need to go into the details here). If, despite your efforts at self-treatment, your attempts to doze off are thwarted by loud "hics," your doctor can order treatment to help you. A few breaths of carbon dioxide or an injection of a sedative medication will generally eliminate the problem.

Backache and Other Aches and Pains

Aches and pains of many types, particularly backaches, are common after surgery. They can be caused by the operation itself. You may lie on a hard operating table, in an unnatural position for several hours; and even though you are asleep, your back and muscles "know" that they've been taxed. The bed rest that follows surgery prevents your joints and muscles from working normally. They become stiff and achy. Strategically placed pillows, a heating pad, moving and changing positions as often as possible and, most important, early exercise are curative. As soon as your doctor and your condition permits it (earlier and earlier these days, often the first night after surgery), you should sit up and dangle your legs, then progress quickly to sitting in a nearby chair, and as soon as possible, walking about.

PRIVATE-DUTY NURSES AND THE POSTSURGICAL PATIENT

We discussed private-duty nurses in Chapter 8. We talked about certain problems for the critically ill patient that private nurses might create. For the routine postsurgical patient the story is quite different. A private nurse, particularly one who has experience with postoperative patients, can be a godsend in the first two or three days after surgery. She can help you deal with all of the discomforts outlined above. She can speed your pain shot and discuss any changes in orders with the nurses or doctor. If she has been around awhile, she may have some special tricks up her sleeve to help you with various discomforts. Most importantly she provides a helping hand at a time when you may feel helpless. She can assist you to shift positions or to move around. She can reach the television control that slipped from your grasp onto the floor. She can bring the magazine from across the room or hand you the telephone that you can't reach yourself. In short, she is a valuable assistant during your brief period of physical impairment.

The problem is that private nurses are quite expensive: approximately two thousand dollars weekly for twenty-four-hour RN coverage, somewhat less for an LPN or nursing aide. Moreover, that expense is your own since very few insurance policies pay for private nurses. You may find that a compromise works well for you. Perhaps you can have family members with you for most of the day and require a private nurse only from 8:00 P.M. to 8:00 A.M. And, since the first few days are the roughest, you may decide to employ a nurse for only two to four days. If you have an LPN for the first four nights following your surgery, the bill will be approximately four hundred dollars.

❦

ASSISTING WITH YOUR RECOVERY

How fast and how well you recover depends to a great extent on you. The harder you work, the faster you'll be up, around, and out. Self-help doesn't merely speed your recovery, it can stave off certain complications.

Thrombophlebitis (blood clots in the veins) is one complication that can occur in bedridden individuals. Your postsurgery efforts can markedly lessen the likelihood of your developing this. Your doctor will want to get your legs moving as soon as possible. He may have you sit up on the first evening after surgery and will try, if your condition permits it, to have you out of bed, in a chair, then walking within a day. An in-bed exercise plan used by many of our surgical colleagues is very beneficial. Simply press your feet against the footboard of the bed and wiggle your toes. Do this for one minute, followed by a rest of one minute, and repeat three times. Try to carry out this easy exercise program every hour or two. The simple act of toe wiggling stimulates muscle activity in your legs, helps pump the blood out of your veins, and decreases the chances of clotting.

Coughing, deep breathing, and fully expanding your lungs is a major deterrent to postoperative pneumonia and other lung complications. The nurses will encourage you to cough and deep-breathe. Your doctor may order IPPB (intermittent positive pressure breathing), a technique that uses a breathing machine to assist you to take the deepest breaths possible. Another excellent method to prevent lung complications is to blow up balloons. Balloon blowing pays two dividends: you help yourself to prevent lung problems; you delight your children, grandchildren, or youngsters on the pediatric unit (the recipients of your labor). Recently a surgeon friend of ours prescribed this exercise to an elderly postsurgical patient. By the end of the day the man's room resembled a circus—at least two hundred brightly colored balloons decorated every corner. Later, with assistance, he traveled down the hall and cheered up twenty sick children with his gifts.

Coughing, deep breathing, IPPB, blowing up balloons can be quite uncomfortable if you've just had abdominal or chest surgery. We gave some useful advice earlier—splint your incision with pillows, and time your exercises thirty minutes after your pain shot.

The greater your determination, the more you work at getting up and around, the faster you'll be home. At times it isn't easy to get out of bed or to cough on command. But we can assure you the ultimate reward is well worth any discomfort. The doctors and nurses can take you a certain distance. You have to walk the final mile.

A GUIDE TO VARIOUS OPERATIONS

SURGERY	* ANESTHESIA	** TIME IN HOSPITAL	*** TIME OUT OF WORK
		(days)	(weeks)
Appendectomy (simple)	G,S	5	2
Appendectomy (ruptured)	G,S	10	4
Cataract extraction (standard)	L,G	4	2
Cataract extraction (phaco)	L,G	2	1
Cesarean section	S,G	5	2
Colon resection (partial)	G,S	12	4
Colon resection (with ileostomy)	G,S	16	6
Coronary artery bypass	G	14	6
Duodenal ulcer (vagotomy and antrectomy)	G	9	3
Gallbladder removal (simple)	G	6	2
Gallbladder removal (with bile duct exploration)	G	12	4
Hernia repair (first time, inguinal)	G,S,L	6	2
Hemorrhoidectomy	S,G	4	2
Hysterectomy (simple)	G,S	6	3
Hysterectomy (with tubes and ovaries removed)	G,S	8	3½
Gastrectomy (partial)	G	9	3
Face lift	L,G	3	3
Knee cartilage (meniscectomy)	S,G	5	2
Laminectomy (lumbar with fusion)	G,S	10	5
Mastectomy (simple)	G	5	2
Mastectomy (radical)	G	7	3
Prostatectomy (transurethral)	S,G	5	2
Prostatectomy (open)	G,S	10	3
Rhinoplasty	G,L	4	2
Tonsillectomy	G	4	2
Tubal ligation (laparoscopic)	S,G	2	1
Thyroidectomy	G	7	2
Vasectomy	L,S,G	2	½

* G *(general)*, S *(spinal)*, L *(local*—often assisted with sedation). Choices are ordered according to usual preferred methods. Each surgeon has his own preference; certain patients may be better off with one form rather than another—i.e., one might choose spinal (if possible) in an elderly patient, rather than general.

** These numbers all represent days. They are merely averages. It should be clearly understood that duration of hospital stays varies markedly, depending upon preferences of the surgeon, progress the patient makes, the age and general health of patient.

*** Also these numbers (weeks) vary widely depending upon nature of job—heavy physical labor versus sedentary—and individual patient progress and response.

14

Special Care Units:
What They Can Do for You
and What You Can Do for a Loved One

Ted, aged nineteen, collided at 50 mph with a concrete bridge abutment; he sustained multiple severe injuries. Soon after admission to the local rural hospital his lungs filled with fluid, threatening to cut off his air exchange. At about the same time he lapsed into a coma. Since he could not receive the necessary critical care at his community hospital, he was transferred by helicopter to the medical center special care unit one hundred miles away.

On admission to the shock-trauma unit, an endotracheal tube (artificial airway) was inserted and attached to a respirator that would do the work of breathing for Ted. He was also hooked up to a cardiac monitor with an assortment of wires. Then an intravenous catheter line was threaded into one of the veins of Ted's left forearm. A plastic tube was attached to this catheter so that Ted could receive continuous regulated sustenance from various bottles of clear fluid hung near the bedside. At the foot of the bed a urinary catheter was draining bloody urine from Ted's bladder into a plastic bag.

Constant nursing attention, aided by electronic monitoring equipment, readily available physician care, and prompt access to the latest drugs and support devices saved Ted's life. After two days he gradually regained consciousness. Within a week he could speak clearly, move his extremities, and begin to sit up. One week later he was out of the trauma unit and well on his way to complete recovery. Ted's story is illustrative of the lifesaving marvels of the modern critical care unit. Ten years ago, Ted would probably have succumbed to his injuries. Today, the availability of this kind of specialized life-support facility kept his vital functions in balance while his system struggled to overcome the injuries.

Time and early support are the hallmarks of the intensive care success story. Each year, thousands of Teds, who only a few years ago would have died, are guided toward full recovery in units like these. In the case of seriously injured patients, intensive care and shock-trauma units have lowered the mortality in some areas from 80 percent to as low as 15 percent. Their cousins—the coronary care units—have improved survival statistics in heart attack victims, reducing mortality in certain groups of patients from a previous 35 percent to a current 16 percent. What makes these statistics even more impressive is that such units have only been around since the early 1960s. They are still in their infant stages of development and hold even greater promise for the future as they are refined and expanded.

∾

THE NEW BREED OF SPECIAL CARE FACILITIES

Technology and modern medical advances gave birth to these and many other kinds of special care units, and their offspring have multiplied and matured. With the proliferation of special care units has come a new group of superspecialized nurses and physicians who are specifically trained to provide skilled management of the patients and conditions that they treat. Today there are many types of special care facilities; some manage and maintain patients with certain illnesses or injuries and others handle particular age groups of patients whose proper care requires highly technical training. Units that care for specific illnesses or injuries include critical care or shock-trauma centers, burn centers, neurological injury units, the more familiar coronary care and intensive care units, and renal dialysis centers. The prototype for the units that care for a special class of patients—in this case determined by age as well as condition—is the neonatal intensive care unit.

Shock-Trauma Centers

Critical care, or shock-trauma, centers are new to the medical scene. Ted, who introduced this chapter, was the fortunate beneficiary of this kind of critical care. In areas (mostly metropolitan) where these have been set up, the mortality rate for victims of serious accidents has dropped dramatically. An ancillary but integral and vital part of the total system is a mechanism for transporting victims from the scene of an accident and the development of sophisticated life-support training for the on-site transport personnel. Several locals have established helivac units (using helicopters) for expeditious transport of the seriously injured. In eastern Maryland, there is a medivac team which can be promptly summoned to the accident scene. The attendants are trained paramedics. They initiate treatment and stay in radio contact with the shock trauma-centers at the University of Maryland Hospital in Baltimore or the Suburban Hospital in Bethesda. They then speed the victim by air to the waiting center where proper intervention—surgical or medical or both—is carried out by an on-call team of trauma specialists. For accidents closer to these centers, the ambulance and rescue squad crews have special training to help manage the accident victim. Many of the ground transportation units also have the sophisticated capability of maintaining a two-way radio dialogue with a physician at the hospital.

The best shock-trauma centers are set up to tap the fullest range of modern medical resources. They have highly skilled nurses and physicians, all of the latest monitoring equipment, immediate access to a wide range of laboratory facilities, a complete complement of life-support machines, and ready access to on-call specialists in every possible field of medicine—general surgery, anesthesiology, urology, neurosurgery, pediatrics, internal medicine as well as the newly recognized field of intensive care (a discipline specifically geared to evaluate and provide ongoing supervision for victims of serious injuries).

Burn Centers

Burn centers, as the name implies, are geared to care for the very special needs of the seriously burned patient. These, too, are relatively new, and although they are available in most major urban areas, smaller rural hospitals cannot support this type of special care unit. However they can and often do make arrangements to evacuate patients by ambulance or helicopter to the nearest center when it is clear that survival depends upon this kind of skilled care. Burn units, too, have dramatically reduced mortality and morbidity (later complications) in patients who receive major burns.

Neurological Injury Units

Neurological injury units are less common than shock-trauma centers. Although many shock-trauma centers handle the full scope of injuries, including head injuries, certain hospitals have established specialized units that care for patients whose primary life-threatening injuries involve the brain and/or spinal cord. Here neurologists, intensivists, neurosurgeons, and specialized nurses attend to the very special needs of the recently paralyzed, the patient in coma, and the patient with bleeding inside his head who may require surgical exploration to remove the blood and control the hemorrhaging.

Intensive Care Units (ICUs)

The intensive care unit (ICU) is, at this point, the oldest and best established of these critical care facilities. Almost every hospital has one, but (as we saw in Chapters 2 and 3) the quality is quite variable, depending upon the expertise of the nurses and whether qualified physicians are always available. These units were established to answer a need for the hospitalized patient. They give a level of care, monitoring, observation, and moment-to-moment treatment changes that regular hospital floors simply cannot provide. They manage patients whose precarious status requires this kind of eagle-eye supervision. The kinds of problems handled here are as varied as medicine itself: patients in shock, recent stroke victims, patients with heart failure, patients with serious infections, individuals with touch-and-go respiratory impairment, and patients who have just undergone extremely major surgical procedures, to name a few. In hospitals that do not have a shock-trauma unit the intensive care unit serves this function—victims of serious accidents are brought here. Patients may be sent to the intensive care unit directly from an emergency department, or they may be transferred there from another section of the hospital or from the postoperative recovery room. Many hospitals have now further subdivided intensive care units into medical and surgical units. Whether the patient goes to the medical intensive care unit (MICU) or the surgical intensive care unit (SICU) depends upon the nature of his illness or injury.

The advent of the ICU was a big step forward in twentieth-century medicine. Together with an ever-expanding array of monitoring and supportive equipment and a supply of the most up-to-date drugs, with new drugs added almost daily, the ICUs help people who used to be beyond help and give remarkable hope for recovery to patients who twenty years ago would surely have died.

Coronary Care Units (CCUs)

The coronary care units (CCU) may be the most familiar of all the special care facilities. They are an offshoot of the ICU and have grown in popularity only in the past ten years. Their rise to prominence has been meteoric. Ten years ago very few hospitals had them. Even an excellent center like the Johns Hopkins University Hospital in Baltimore had no CCU in 1968. Now, only the tiniest of the seven thousand hospitals in this country lack a CCU. And most of those hospitals that have CCUs have at least a few nurses who are specifically trained to evaluate and manage heart attack victims.

The CCU, particularly in major centers, has improved survival statistics for the heart attack sufferer. But the results are not as striking as those in the ICU or the shock-trauma centers. In fact, some authorities on health care costs are currently questioning the need for a unit in every hospital. They point to the data and claim that the small reduction in heart attack deaths isn't worth the

A main problem in saving individuals stricken by heart attacks is that the majority who are going to die do so before they reach the hospital. That's why many large cities have developed sophisticated paramedic transport teams who can speed to the victim's side in a minute. As an adjunct to the CCU, these teams are adding an extra measure of success. The rescue personnel are trained in cardiopulmonary resuscitation (CPR), and many have two-way communications with the hospital emergency department and/or the CCU and can even transmit, by phone, the patient's electrocardiogram. Armed with the relevant clinical data, a doctor at the other end can radio back instructions, thereby reducing the loss of vital time while the patient is on route to the hospital. These paramedic teams in combination with the CCU (which may eventually become centralized rather than located in every hospital) offer new hope for heart attack victims.

Renal Dialysis Centers

Renal dialysis centers are a form of special care unit. But unlike the others we discussed, they are not designed to manage acutely ill patients or to combat a brief life-threatening episode. Instead, they serve a chronic care function. They provide the artificial kidneys for patients whose kidneys have stopped functioning. The dialysis unit differs in another important respect from other special care facilities. Because it serves long-term needs for individuals who have returned to society, it provides care for outpatients as well as patients within the hospital. Renal dialysis and renal transplantation offer a great hope for victims of kidney disease. Many who would have died twenty years ago can now live active and productive lives.

Neonatal Intensive Care Units (NICUs)

The neonatal intensive care unit specializes, as the name indicates, in problems of the newborn. Instead of dividing patients into disease groups—the CCU for heart attack victims, the dialysis unit for those stricken by kidney disease, the shock-trauma center for the acutely injured—it accepts newborns with all sorts of serious illnesses. The reason for this division is very simple. Newborns present special management problems. It takes very skilled nursing and physician care to deal with these diminutive people. Their fluid requirements, temperature control, oxygen management, drugs are all different from standard adult needs. These units have given even the tiniest of premature infants a new lease on life. They have changed the survival statistics dramatically so that today even a two-pound infant, with ideal care, has a reasonable chance of surviving.

THE FAMILY'S ROLE IN HELPING PATIENTS IN SPECIAL CARE UNITS

Transient psychiatric problems have been reported by special care unit personnel from all over the world. The "intensive care syndrome" and "postcardiotomy delirium" are new diseases of "medical progress." In one series of ninety adult open-heart procedures, 40 percent of the patients were described as delirious sometime during the first three postoperative days as compared to less than 1 percent of patients undergoing other types of operations. Similar happenings are indigenous to the CCU and medical ICU. As one observer described, "The patient might first experience a perceptual distortion; for example, the sound arising from the air-conditioning vent might begin to sound like his name." In some patients these distortions of reality progressed to the point of auditory or visual hallucinations and then to frank paranoid delusions. In cases involving the ICU or CCU the mental disturbances slowly evolved after a lucid period of roughly three to five days. Usually this psychosis cleared within twenty-four to forty-eight hours following transfer to the standard hospital environment.

Some psychiatrists suggest that this emotional disturbance is a close first cousin to the more well-known "sensory deprivation syndrome." The critically ill patient is in an environment that is constantly lit and frequently devoid of windows, thus day and night are indistinguishable. The major field of vision consists of panels of acoustic tile and fluorescent lighting fixtures. People sounds are muffled by buzzes, hums, and clicks from the life-support systems. Personnel cannot dally for more than a few kind words of encouragement, and often they become callous and unsupportive emotionally. Physical touching is limited to bed or equipment adjustments. Brief family visits by obviously frightened loved ones do not normally provide necessary reassurance.

What can be done to alleviate the emotional deterioration that special care units can bring? Some units have addressed this problem by adding a psychiatric social worker to the team. We also like the concept of a medically unsophisticated patient ombudsman, who will hold the patient's hand, discuss the news and weather, and support the patient emotionally.

You, as a family member, should make your very brief visits substantive, positive, and pleasant. Don't ask "Are you in pain?" Instead recite the latest ball scores. Keep the patient in touch with as much pleasant reality as possible. If the patient cannot respond because of a tracheostomy tube or an altered state of consciousness, don't ask questions! Read him the funnies!

Direct your contribution toward taking the patient's mind off the artificial environment. A touch of home and a warm familiar embrace provide a remarkable tonic for these otherwise medically imprisoned individuals. In special care units familiarity breeds content.

15

Some Practical Answers
to Questions About
Daily Hospital Life

There are many nuances of hospital life that are important to patients but don't specifically relate to nursing or physician care. The following are some of the daily activities and the creature comforts that can make for a more or less pleasant hospital experience: visitors, roommates, phone calls, television, patient orientation, food, special patient education, bookmobiles, arts and crafts services, having spouses sleep in, and even the seemingly mundane matter of gifts from visitors.

cﾞﾟﾟ

VISITORS AND VISITING HOURS

One of the most common patient complaints deals with visitors—too many or, at the other extreme, hours that are too brief. Obviously the number of visitors and frequency of visitations must be directly related to two things: how sick the patient is and the patient's personal desires.

Patients who are recovering from surgery, a severe heart attack, or a critical illness need rest. They don't need a constant parade of visitors with whom they have to converse. Patients like these frequently complain about being worn out by too many visitors. They have the distinct feeling that they are the hosts or hostesses, and they are, therefore, obliged to entertain their friends and relatives: a burden that no patient should have to bear. The most striking example of this occurs when a physician is hospitalized in his own hospital. He will frequently be inundated by physicians, nurses, orderlies, and other co-workers, in addition to the usual family and friends. We have actually seen a case of a physician friend whose recovery from a heart attack was severely impaired by this flow of well-wishers.

Too many visitors can interfere with patient care in other ways. We have seen patients refuse to go for their X-rays because a group of friends were visiting. We have seen patients in the next bed complain about the disturbance created by visitors across the room.

What can the patient or family members do to control the number of visitors or phone calls (another source of disruption)? You may request "no information." The request is made to the nurse. This means that if anyone calls to inquire about you, the operator will not give out any information. You are, in this manner, able to keep your whereabouts private. Visitors can only come if you or a relative invite them. Similarly, you can arrange for the hospital operator not to put any call through to your room. Only those who know the direct dial line can get through.

You may wish to limit visitation to immediate family only. Some hospitals provide for this by issuing passes to predetermined visitors. No one without a pass is permitted to visit.

We realize that some individuals—those well on their way to recovery, those who are in the hospital for a chronic problem like traction for fracture management, or people who simply can't stand being alone—may want to have visitors. This is fine as long as there aren't so many of them that they disturb neighbors, interfere with the therapeutic program, or break the hospital's visiting rules.

A close family member may want and need to stay with a relative to assist with special needs and creature comforts. This is somewhat different from the visitation situation discussed above.

An elderly stroke victim may need the comfort and physical help that her daughter can offer. A frightened child must have as much contact as possible with his parents. In a sense, these are not really visitors. They are contributors to the patient's recovery program. What they must realize (and we believe that most close relatives do) is that their loved ones need to sleep and require peace and quiet. The helpful relative is there when he or she is needed but sits quietly in the background or goes out for something to eat when his sick relative shows signs of tiring.

Most hospitals have specific visiting hours and a limit of two visitors per patient. The rules vary from hospital to hospital and from floor to floor. Often private floors are less strict about visiting rules. The hours may be broader and more flexible, and the number of visitors allowed may be greater. However, even private patients need their rest. Parades of visitors can interfere with their smooth recovery as well.

ॐ

ROOMMATES VERSUS PRIVATE ROOM: HOW DO YOU CHOOSE?

Decision number one: Do you want a roommate? Private rooms are generally available, although they may require an advance reservation. The determining factors are primarily personal and financial. Do you prefer to be alone? Can you afford the extra daily expense?

You may cherish your privacy, have business or other work to carry on and, therefore, need to be undisturbed. If so, opt for a private room.

There are a few advantages of being with someone else which might not be immediately obvious. In many cases we have seen patients change their minds after a few days of isolation. They found the loneliness of a private room unpleasant and preferred to share their hospital experience with a neighbor. For elderly, confused, or infirm patients, an alert roomate can be a real asset. Roommates often become quite protective of their sicker or less-in-touch neighbors. They help them. They'll call the nurse when an elderly roommate drops his call button, warn a neighbor not to get out of bed without assistance when he shouldn't be doing so, yell for help when an acute crisis occurs in the next bed. For these patients who don't have family members or private-duty nurses around and who may need physical assistance, roommates can be quite useful.

Roommates can also be obstreperous, annoying, a real detriment to recovery. They may smoke when you can't stand smoke. They may have oxygen running which prevents you from smoking when you want to. They may snore or make other unpleasant noises. They may have noisy, frequent visitors. They may inconsiderately watch television late into the night. If you are "so blessed," having a roommate can be a real drag.

If your situation is intolerable, you can ask for a change. The reason has to be a pretty good one, not one that is frivolous or that is easily corrected by a calm discussion. The reason that changes can't be made at will, for minimal complaints, is because they are troublesome and costly. Approximately twenty different hospital facilities must be notified: the admitting office, the switchboard, the laboratory, the X-ray department, the kitchen, etc. In addition, a few days' worth of records—X-ray reports, laboratory slips, and other studies—are often lost when patients are transferred. You might ask, "Why can't they simply be forwarded?" They can be, but the fact of the matter is that they often aren't. It is estimated that a room switch costs the hospital between one and two hundred dollars in time and mechanical changes. And loss of important patient data can be hazardous. So if you must change rooms, tell the nurse. You'll probably be able to do so if another room is available. However, if possible, try to correct your problem without moving elsewhere.

PATIENT ORIENTATION

The nurses or the patient representative will generally give the patient some general hospital information when he arrives on the floor, or a packet may be handed out in the admitting office. This includes delineation of visiting hours, availability of televisions and how to get them, information about bookmobile services and other patient activity resources, visitor eating facilities and patient lounges. In addition, the nurse should instruct the patient regarding the floor personnel—who the various people are and what they do—and the call system. Today there is usually a nurses' call button at the bedside and an intercom at the nurses' station. When the patient calls the nurse asks, by intercom, what the patient wants. If the patient doesn't respond promptly, suggesting a possible serious problem, the nurse should come running. An urgent verbal summons from the patient should elicit the same response. More minor matters, like fresh ice water, are taken care of when the nursing staff has time.

Occasionally the nurses forget to provide proper instructions to patients, or they may not realize that an elderly senile individual or stroke victim may not understand. A vital service that a close relative can and must perform is to be certain that his loved one is able to get help when he or she needs it. The button must be situated in a reachable place and not on the side of a paralyzed arm. It is advisable that the friend or relative bringing the patient in be certain that the patient knows where the call button is and how to use it. You might even ask him to demonstrate once to be sure, before he is left alone.

HOSPITAL FOOD

A few hospitals, probably as a protest against the usual grumblings about tasteless hospital food, have overreacted. They serve gourmet delicacies ranging from steak Diane to lobster Thermidor. Their extensive mouth-watering menus would seem far more at home at the Four Seasons restaurant than at Glenwood General. But don't start smacking your lips and impatiently counting the days until your planned hospitalization, for the chances are only four or five out of seven thousand that your hospital will offer that kind of fare.

Most often, hospital food isn't exciting or delectable. Institutional, large-volume food preparation is not conducive to fine cooking. Storing the food after it is prepared, carrying it up several floors, and delivering it to hundreds of patients further compromises its appeal: hot things become cool, ice cream melts, and meat that may have started out moist dries out.

The responsibility of the food preparation team is, in this order: to provide patients their proper medically indicated diets; to prepare well-balanced, nourishing meals; to offer a broad enough selection to satisfy most tastes; and (unfortunately last) to make the food appetizing and tasty. Not that the last isn't important, it is simply the hardest to accomplish.

The taste-pleasing (or displeasing) quality of hospital food varies markedly from institution to institution, depending upon the abilities of the cooks and the nature of the food transport services. Today hospital food is generally acceptable except to the most finicky or discriminating eater. Most important, the quality of the food is usually excellent, and the staff of well-trained professional dietary personnel see to it that it is medically correct, well balanced, and nourishing.

The most important food advice we can give you is to be sure to avoid any major dietary errors. If you are eating regular foods without restrictions, this doesn't apply to you. But if you are on a strict salt-free diet, let the nurse know if you are delivered the corned beef intended for your next-door neighbor. Or if you have had an abdominal operation and have just started drinking liquids, question the roast beef and mashed potato dinner that you are served. The diet service or the food transporters can make mistakes, so be sure to inquire if you know that the food is wrong for you or if you aren't quite sure.

If you find a particular meal unpalatable, tell your nurse as soon as possible. At times they can make a change to something else. If all of the meals are inedible, you have a problem, for it is unlikely that the kitchen can be modified to suit you. However, if the problem is one that can probably be corrected, such as the food always being too cold, you may be able to change that. Ask the nurse to have one of the dieticians visit you to discuss your dissatisfaction. Even if it's a difficulty that cannot be corrected immediately, it is important that the food service be informed of food complaints. They do have some obligation to try to please, and in general, they want to. They must be made aware of food preparation and food transporting shortcomings.

You may not be aware of the fact that you may be able to have food brought in from the outside. Unless there is some specific contraindication to this, because of a special diet for instance, there is usually no objection to having a friend or relative bring you a hamburger or even a pizza. An occasional meal from outside can break up the monotony of hospital food. If you simply cannot tolerate the food the hospital serves you, you may even be able to have most of your meals delivered from a relative's kitchen or a nearby takeout eatery.

If you check into the hospital late in the day, there are sometimes problems getting your first meal. The kitchen requires some notice to prepare it for you. If you hope to have dinner served that first night, you should ask the nurse as soon as you arrive to order it for you.

The nurses generally have some snack-type foods available on the floor. If you are hungry before bedtime, you may be able to get some jello, pudding, ice cream, cookies, milk, or other fillers to satisfy your late-night cravings.

e&

SPECIAL PATIENT EDUCATION

In recent years, hospitals have paid more and more attention to patient education. They recognize the need to inform their patients, and they are responding to this new awareness. The types of programs available are quite variable. They include booklets and pamphlets, descriptive video-tape and slide presentations that may be brought into the patient's room or may take place (for those patients who are mobile) in central viewing areas, visits from special education personnel, and even closed-circuit TV programs piped into each patient's room and viewable on the regular television set. Educational programs may include information about various operative procedures, general information about hospital services and personnel, discussions of how to deal with problems that may arise, presentations about caring for a new baby, and many other programs of general and specific interest. Since hospitals vary greatly with regard to these services, it is best to ask the floor nurse, when you are admitted, whether any such program of particular interest to you is available in the hospital.

❦

BOOKMOBILES AND ARTS AND CRAFTS SERVICES

Most hospitals have bookmobiles and arts and crafts services. The latter may be brought to the patient's room, or the ambulatory patient may go to an arts and crafts center. Not every patient is physically able to participate in these activities, and some patients may simply not wish to. But for many patients in the recuperative phases of their illnesses or in the hospital for diagnostic testing, these diversions afford an excellent way of whiling away otherwise tedious hours.

❦

RELATIVES SLEEPING IN

In some hospital settings a relative can, and may even be encouraged to, share the room with his or her loved one. This is particularly common in children's hospitals where children undergoing elective surgery can often have mom or dad spend the night. The accommodations may not be plush, often a daybed or a hideaway sleeper of some sort, but the discomfort is well worth it. Children especially are far less frightened if a parent stays with them. If your child is about to be hospitalized, we would encourage you to check whether this service is available. If so, take advantage of it.

Adults can sometimes stay with spouses, in private rooms of course. Some hospitals offer this, many do not. If it is available, whether or not you chose to go that route depends upon personal preference and how much help the patient needs.

❧

GIFTS

You've all experienced a hospital room so loaded with plants, flowers, baskets of fruit that it looks like a combination arboretum-orchard. Whether or not gifts like these are practical and worthwhile is more a matter of opinion and philosophy than fact. Showing your concern for a sick friend or relative by sending a gift is a nice gesture. The advice that we can offer is to choose a gift wisely. Don't send flowers to an asthmatic who may be allergic to them. Don't send candy to someone who has just undergone stomach surgery. A gift that will last, like a plant, is generally well received. Consider the possibility of deferring the gift until the patient returns home. Patients who require some home convalescence are generally forgotton once they leave the hospital. The flow of presents stops abruptly.

Some special care areas and even certain hospital floors restrict gifts or ban them altogether. Coronary care units, intensive care units, burn wards cannot be cluttered with gifts. Pulmonary care units which care for patients with breathing disorders will generally not permit any plants or flowers. Thus, before sending a gift, be sure that the intended recipient is permitted to accept it.

If you arrive with a gift and realize that it is inappropriate—the patient with a tube in his nose can't even look at the candy, the room is so cluttered with flowers that another bouquet would be overwhelming, there is a sign requesting "no gifts please"—a good alternative is to give the gift to the nurses in the name of the patient. Let the patient know that you are doing this. The nurses will appreciate the gesture.

A rewarding gift that is usually appreciated by patients who can see and function is something which can occupy their time: a novel, a crossword puzzle book, a game, indicates special thought and consideration. We recommend giving gifts like these. If you know the patient well, take a moment to consider his special interests. Personalize a gift by making it something particularly apropos.

16

Preparing Your Child for the Hospital

"She's having too many ear infections; fluid is collecting behind the drums again. We'll get her over this infection with antibiotics —*again,* but we've got to prevent recurrences or her ears will be permanently damaged. We've discussed this before; we'll have to operate," your pediatrician informs you.

You knew that was coming as soon as Lisa started crying and holding her ear last night. You dreaded hearing the word "operate," yet you were anticipating it, bracing yourself for it all night long. Well, he said it; now we begin the planning: the when, where, and how.

"What does *operate* mean, Mommy?" asks Lisa. "Can I still get my lollipop?"

Involved with your own fears and expectations, you realize that you have given little thought to deciding how you would explain all of this to little, trusting Lisa. Suddenly all of the arrangements seem less important than how you will present this new, frightening, painful adventure to your five-year-old. With some relief you note that you have some time to think about it and discuss it with Lisa.

You look at the bruised and bleeding leg, horribly swollen and deformed, and then at the tearful, pained face of your two-year-old son. It's clear that he has had a serious leg injury. He will have to be hospitalized so that the bone can be surgically aligned and casted. The doctor wants him to be sedated and medicated as soon as possible so that surgery can begin. Little time is left: What can you or should you say to him when he cries out and reaches for you to hold him and take him home?

A child who needs to be hospitalized presents a challenge to his parents, his doctor, the hospital, and its staff. Naturally we want to protect the child and prepare him as well as possible for this experience. Children, after all, are special people whose world is inhabited by powerful adults, fantasy dreams, monsters, unknowns. A trip through childhood is one in which the unknowns become knowns and the monsters tamed.

Our job as adults is to take the fear out of the unknown, simplify the complex world of the hospital, and explain the potentially frightening events to come for our children. If your child is to be hospitalized for an *elective* procedure, an operation, or diagnostic studies, both you and your child are fortunate: you have the luxury of time to prepare for the new, complex, and possibly difficult experiences your child will face.

❧

YOUR OWN PREPARATION FOR YOUR CHILD'S HOSPITALIZATION

In order to allay your child's fears, first you'll have to overcome some of your own. Prepare by making the unfamiliar, familiar; the unexpected, anticipated. Although you cannot anticipate every event, at least by making important events familiar you and your child will be better prepared.

If your child must be admitted for an elective hospitalization, you both have a lot to learn and understand. Ask your child's doctor the following questions:

· When is the admission date and time?

· What should you bring besides pajamas, toothbrush, and the other obvious things that common sense dictates? (Try to think of some favorite, familiar things to make your child's bed a comforting spot in an alien world: a personal toy, stuffed animal, activity tools, crafts, or a favorite storybook.

· Will you be able to bring a favorite treat—gum, candy, cookies—the night before or after the procedure?

· What tests will be required (blood, urine, X-rays), and when (on admission or later?), and where (in the patient's room or in the laboratory?), and can you be present?

· What special procedures are scheduled? What do they involve? When are they scheduled? Can you be present?

· If surgery is planned:
1. What anesthetic will be used? How long will it last? Will your child be premedicated in the room or in the operating suite?
2. Can you accompany your child to the operating room area? (Some hospitals have a parent area right outside the operating room suite where you can hold your child's hand until he is asleep.)
3. After surgery how long will your child be asleep? Can you see him in the recovery room when he awakens?
4. How much postoperative pain can he expect?
5. How soon will he be able to eat?
6. What about postoperative activities and restrictions?
7. Will there be any postoperative drains, tubes, etc.?
8. Might private duty nurses be helpful?

· How long will the hospital stay be?

· Can you stay with your child? If not, what are the visiting and phone hours?

· Can you take your child to the hospital on a walking tour of the floors? (Perhaps the child can meet some of the nurses and even see the operating room. Many hospitals can arrange this sort of preadmission preparation for children.)

This list may seem overzealous, but you would be amazed at the questions that both you and your child can think of later and be sorry that you hadn't asked. No question is too trivial. Your child's comfort and peace of mind is ultimately at stake. However, keep in mind that your doctor may not have all the answers. Some of these questions can be dealt with by the office nurse, hospital guides, or any nurses you may meet on a hospital tour.

❦

SELECTING THE HOSPITAL

In general, children's hospitals provide the best, most specialized, and the most complete care for their children patients. They accommodate both of your child's needs: creature comforts and quality care. The nurses and physicians are familiar with the unique needs of children. They have the most sophisticated equipment to handle a child's health problems and the broadest base of pediatric specialists. In addition, they make life most comfortable for their little patients. The decor, the bathroom facilities, the call buttons, the TV, the food, the family lounges, and playrooms are all designed for small people. How comforting for your child to see other children, toys, brightly painted rooms, toilets of the right height, small TVs within reach of the bed, peanut butter and jelly sandwiches on the menu. Such hospitals are more receptive to parents remaining overnight and accompanying the child throughout much of the testing. If you have a choice, opt for a children's hospital.

Second best are hospitals that have pediatric units. They, too, have specialized nurses, a complement of pediatric equipment, and an understanding of children's needs. Frequently they are willing to work with parents to lessen the anxiety of a hospital stay. Many permit parents to room in.

What if your community is too small to offer specialized children's care? What if there are no children's hospitals or separate pediatric facilities? If your child's tonsils need to come out, if he needs a routine orthopedic procedure (setting a broken bone), an appendectomy, or routine eye or ear surgery, these level-two procedures (see Chapter 2) can be performed in most hospitals provided the anesthesia department has appropriate pediatric equipment and experience. Your surgeon or pediatrician should know this and can help you decide whether to remain in town or travel to a pediatric center.

However, should your child require open-heart surgery; close neurological evaluation, and possible neuroradiologic evaluation and neurosurgery (after a concussion or severe head injury, or for a brain tumor or increased pressure inside the head); extensive abdominal surgery (not simply an appendectomy), or should he require an intensive care unit or sophisticated diagnostic work-up, surely you would want the best, most up-to-date care available. The same considerations we suggested in Chapters 2 and 3 concerning finding the best hospital for these problems should also be applied to your choice of a children's facility. Therefore, the first consideration is the quality of care. If your hospital cannot provide the range of health care services your child may need, you should (unless a move is impossible) take him elsewhere.

HOW TO CHANGE YOUR CHILD'S DOCTOR

If you feel that the care afforded at another center is demanded, you may have to change physicians. Depending upon the problem, it is likely that your doctor will recommend such a hospital, be familiar with referral techniques, and provide you with the name of another physician (or physicians). Even if your physician is not completely happy with your desire to go elsewhere, he or she should be willing to recommend a competent physician at another center. It may be difficult for your physician to admit that the local hospital, or that he, is not capable of handling your child's problem. You can facilitate matters by understanding this, just as he will understand that your paramount concern is the child's welfare—you are both, after all, trying to do the best for the sick child.

You may still want this physician to care for your child once this acute problem or diagnostic puzzle is clarified and solved. Hence, getting a referral directly from him is the best approach.

If you meet hostility and resistance, you must have the courage to face the situation and stand up for your convictions. Keep in mind that your doctor cannot ethically just throw up his hands and tell you to do what you will without him. If he feels you cannot work together, he is bound ethically to recommend at least one or two other physicians to you. If you are still dissatisfied, you can call the pediatric center nearest you and speak with the specific department under whose care your child would be. Find out the name of the chief of the service and see whether he or she or another member of the department (whom the chief could recommend to you) would be willing to accept and care for your child.

◌⅊◌

PREPARING YOUR CHILD FOR A HOSPITAL STAY

Once your doctor has advised you that your child's problem will require an operation or a diagnostic evaluation in the hospital, needless to say, you are concerned. Remember that "hospital," "operation," "tests" are unfamiliar and possibly frightening words to your child. She's probably upset and worried, just as you are.

Some of your fears can be allayed or, at least, controlled by questioning your doctor. Your new knowledge can then be conveyed to your child for the same purpose: to make the unknown, known, thereby removing much of its terror.

Part of the child's fear of the coming hospital stay is related to anger: anger at being taken away from her mother and father, anger at the possible intrusion into her body, anger at the thought of pain. As a sympathetic adult you should accept these emotions, explain to the child that she will be returning home and let her know that it's reasonable and acceptable to feel frightened and angry. It's no help at all to flatly state, "There's nothing to be afraid of." Both you and your child know that's not true.

The easiest way to explain the upcoming hospitalization is in a forthright fashion, assuming your child is at least three years old and can understand. The first explanation will come from the doctor or, perhaps, from both of you jointly, "Your heart is sick, and it's making you feel tired all of the time. It needs to be fixed." "Your eye is crooked, and the doctor will make it straight." Sometimes it is difficult to be matter-of-fact with a small child, but, as a rule, an honest straightforward approach is the least frightening and the best way for your child to get the news.

Some children have dolls or wooden people. It may be helpful to encourage your child to play a hospital game. You can act out some of the tests, the operation, the bandaging, with her using her toys. This tends to bring a new and strange experience into her own familiar world. It also brings out hidden fears, ones that she may not be able to express directly. "How will my dolly be able to go to the bathroom with all those bandages on?" "Poor dolly, she won't have any insides left." It is easy to realize that "dolly" means "me" and your child is telling you what concerns she has.

Children have vivid imaginations that supply explanations for what's happening to them. There may be misinterpretations of what they see or hear. They know their heart is sick or their tonsils are infected. "Will the doctor take my heart out and put a new one in?" "If I lose my tonsils, will I still be able to eat or talk?" "If my eye is crooked, does he have to take it out to operate on it? Will I be able to see afterwards?" The attentive parent hears what the child is saying and can deal with those concerns.

Have your child explain to you what she understands about her coming hospitalization—either through storytelling, drawing, or "people" play. You will soon unravel her fears, misconceptions, and confusions. Then, direct, simplified clarifications can reduce her worries. Always be truthful, not overly detailed, but truthful. We always shudder when we hear parents consoling their screaming children, "Don't worry, the shot won't hurt a bit." Of course it will hurt! Not much, perhaps, but it will hurt. The parent who deceives his child like that will never again be trusted. Children are wonderfully candid. If only the adults around them would be the same way.

Keep your promises to a minimum; many of the things that will happen will hurt, so don't lie about pain. Tell your child that some tests may hurt, but they won't last long—all true. Let him know that you'll be sleeping in the room with him or, if this is not the case, that you will visit frequently. There will be other children to meet and play with when he's up to playing. Most reassuring of all, let your child know that soon he will be coming home again.

No amount of honesty, explanation, and reassurance will remove all of the unknowns. Some of our suggestions will help. These, coupled with a tour of the hospital, will go a long way toward smoothing the actual admission.

On the day prior to admission, if the child is old enough, you might allow him to pack. Let him pick a few of his favorite things— a transistor radio can be a good companion and, if he is old enough to make calls, a list of important phone numbers plus a pencil and pad for his bedside.

A small child will be the most disoriented and frightened. She may not respond to any verbal consolation, but may only be comforted by being held. However, don't forget that more grown-up adolescents and teen-agers will be frightened too. Their concerns may be expressed more directly to you but may also be couched in hostility and anger. The nursing personnel frequently bear the brunt of this adolescent hostility.

Again, honesty with questions and answers, anticipation and understanding of fears will help him to trust you and the other adults who will be caring for him. Depending upon your child's age, he may want to question the doctor directly and privately. Encourage that. He has a right to be as informed a patient as you, yourself, would like to be.

THE CHILD IN THE HOSPITAL

Upon admission to the hospital and more specifically to the floor, both your child and you will have the opportunity to learn the inside workings of the hospital and the floor from the nurses. In addition, and at least as important, you will have the chance of actually determining major portions of your child's treatment and hospital schedule. Thus, the admission interview with the floor nurse provides a vital exchange of information. All of the nurses involved in your child's care will refer to the care plan designed from the information you provide the interviewing nurse.

If the hospital is one of the thousands around the country which is making the change from traditional to "primary care nursing," the nurse you meet first and talk with on admission will be the primary nurse caring for your child throughout his stay. This nurse will be the one whom you work with to make the hospitalization as comfortable and comforting as possible. This knowledge should be reassuring to you and your child; to know that each day will not bring an ever-changing parade of nurses whom you and your child do not know, or who do not know either of you. Thus, each day will not be like starting anew: the same inquiries will not have to be answered again or the same fears reexplained. You have the comfort of a familiar face, the understanding of a knowing professional who has been with you since admission.

The primary nurse will interview both you and your child to gather the most complete profile yet compiled by any health care professional. Its purpose is to design a very individual and personal treatment plan tailored to that unique individual—your child. Primary nursing care plans are comprehensive: detailing usual hours of rising, going to sleep, favorite activities, favorite television programs, likes and dislikes. They generally include a discussion of anticipated tests (dates and times), scheduled surgery, pre- and postoperative medications, permitted activities, and expected physical limitations and capabilities during the stay. It is often here that you learn the "nitty-gritty" of hospital life. This is obviously a valuable interview, and a time when you and your child (if he is old enough) can put your personal touches on the nursing care plan. This is the time to tell the nurse about the favorite worn teddy bear, the night light, or the intolerance to milk.

If your hospital is of the traditional type rather than one that has moved to the primary care system, you will still have an admission interview wth a nurse. Although the information she gathers may not be as comprehensive as described above, clearly she will ask you for the kinds of things medically vital and those things the nurses will need to know in order to help the staff adapt the hospital routine and requirements to your child. In this type of interview more of the burden will be placed upon you, as parents, to supplement what is asked with those things you know to be important: food likes and dislikes (probably more important to a child than an adult patient), bed wetting, favorite TV programs. Keep in mind that the medically vital information will be asked, but the more personal things may require your taking the lead. One other difference from the primary care plan is that there is not necessarily one nurse who will greet you and be with you thereafter, either to plan the recovery goals and anticipated levels of activities postoperatively or to learn and then assimilate the personalized information you provide into her approach to your child's care. This is not to say that traditional nurses don't try to provide warm, personalized care, that skilled medical and surgical care isn't provided, or that traditional nursing care plans don't attempt to take into account some unique features of your child's personality. It is simply that primary care nursing is specifically designed to improve upon the hospital's traditional methods of nursing, maintaining all of its strengths and expanding the role of the nurse in order to provide the patient with a consistent, familiar, concerned professional who directly contributes to the care and recovery plan.

⊷⊷

EMERGENCY ADMISSIONS

Of course not all hospitalizations are elective: acute infections, sudden injuries, appendicitis, poisonings demand emergency hospitalization. Some will follow an office visit to your child's doctor; others will take place through the emergency department of the hospital. Depending upon the severity of the problem, your child may or may not be fully aware of the events happening to him. However, sooner or later he will become aware of the unfamiliar surroundings.

There is little, other than usual maternal or paternal soothing, that you can do to mollify your screaming infant, your vomiting toddler, or your feverish aching adolescent as they face hospitalization. Sometimes your child is too young to understand or too sick to try. For very little children, the best you can do is simply to be with them. Your presence and your comforting familiar voice will help soothe them. If your child is confined to a restricted unit—an intensive care unit for example—simply visit as much as you are permitted to. Your presence is particularly helpful during mealtimes, X-ray procedures, painful tests, or when medications are given.

HELPING YOUR CHILD RECOVER

As your child begins to feel better, the healing process will go more rapidly if you learn the hospital routine and the treatment schedule and explain them to your sick offspring. The knowledge of what lies ahead, how long it will take, and when it will end will define the illness and make it a concrete, finite event for the youngster.

When you understand the treatment protocol, you benefit your child in another way. You are able to monitor the care delivered. If you understand the plan, you won't let your child eat on the morning before an operation. If you know that he is supposed to be eating only clear liquids, you will put your hand out to stop the steak dinner that arrives on his tray. An informed parent can prevent erroneous tests or wrong medications from being administered. Naturally there will be times when you were not informed that a new medication or test was ordered. There is no harm in asking the nurse to check the order sheets to be certain there is no mistake.

An important aspect of illness is the recovery period. Often an observant parent can tell that things are better or that something is amiss earlier and more accurately than the physician can. The first sign of infection is listlessness and vague discomfort, which parents can read very effectively in their children. Most good children's doctors, realizing that parents have this special knack, take parental observations very seriously. If your child changes from day to day and seems to be declining or not doing well, tell his doctor.

At the end of the hospital stay, some healing—both psychological and physical—may need to take place at home. You might want to take pictures during the hospital stay or have the child keep a diary or draw his own impressions. Reviewing and remembering helps to eliminate the subconscious disruption that a traumatic hospital stay can bring. The pictures or written accounts will become an important part of the child's growing-up period. It is his or her story, perhaps painful and unpleasant, but one which must be integrated positively into his future.

Appropriate planning before, adequate comfort and support during, and gentle sympathetic review after the hospital stay are all vital to minimize the negative impact of this event. In fact, if parents perform their roles well, a child's hospital stay can become a very positive, strengthening life experience.

17

Leaving the Hospital

"Al, your cardiogram looks stable now, you're not having any more chest pain, and you seem to be regaining your strength. I'll send you home tomorrow morning. Call your wife and tell her to pick you up about eleven," announces your doctor with a smile.

Al just spent twenty days in the hospital recovering from a heart attack. He's delighted to be going home, so delighted that he simply says, "Thanks, Doc. I really appreciate the care you've given me. See you in the morning!"

It is at this point·that some of the most critical patient-physician communication should take place. If your doctor doesn't initiate it, you should! "What do I do when I get home, Doctor? Is there a special diet that I should be on? Do you want me to lose some more weight? When can I start smoking again? How do I take these drugs you prescribed? Are there any activities I should avoid? When can my wife and I resume our honeymoon? Do you want to see me back in your office soon?"

Ask all those questions now! Better still, ask if there are any written instructions for you to follow during the next several weeks. Some hospitals not only provide written instructions but also will make sure that you have received and understood those instructions by having you sign a statement to that effect.

There are many hospitals that employ nurses whose sole responsibility is to provide patient education. Their task is to make certain that you understand your diet, drugs, activities, and follow-up care. Your job is to pay attention, ask questions until the instructions are clear, then follow the instructions.

Before you actually leave the hospital, there is the matter of the bill. If you have health insurance, a substantial portion of the costs will be covered. You are responsible for the difference between your coverage and the final tally. At discharge the billing office will discuss this reconciliation and require a payment or accept a credit card or send a statement.

REVIEWING THE BILL

We have in front of us a hospital bill. It covered a six-week hospital stay for a desperately ill woman who required three operations and many days of intensive care. The total: $19,300. We learn two things from this bill: how expensive hospital care can be and how difficult it is for anyone, layman or professional, to interpret the many pages listing the hospital charges.

The base daily room charge varies widely from area to area—New York City may be twice as high as Selma, Alabama—but the cost everywhere is high and rising all the time. A semiprivate room costs between $120 and $230 daily, with no extras. That doesn't include any supplies, laboratory studies, or other patient services. Each time the lab technician draws blood from your vein you can expect a bill of from $50 to $300, depending on which tests are performed. Consider how often that happens when you are in the hospital—often once a day—and you've automatically doubled the room charge. A urinalysis is another $25 added to your bill, a chest X-ray another $25 to $50, and a barium enema examination is $100 or more. In the case of drugs you're charged by the pharmacy for every pill, every intravenous bottle, every shot. Bandages, needles, tubing for intravenous bottles, cast materials, and scores of other incidental equipment and supplies are all billed to you by the hospital's central supply department. Other procedures, tests, operations, anesthesia, and special care—private duty nurses, recovery room, ICU, CCU—all cost extra. Suffice it to say that this six-week bill that we are reviewing covers thirty pages. Literally each Band-Aid and each pill has its own line and its own charge.

When you consider hospital costs and hospital bills this way, you can see why costs are so high. You can also see why, except for certain very broad items or the occasional very brief stay, it is impossible to validate completely the accuracy of the bill. You may find two pages that say "Central Supply," with items ranging in cost from one to twenty dollars. These include each individual piece of gauze and adhesive tape used to cover your incision, the splint used for your broken arm, the plaster that formed your leg cast, the disposable mattress cover for your bed, each plastic non-reissuable syringe, etc. The four-page pharmacy section enumerates and prices each pill, tablet, shot, intravenous bottle, teaspoon of milk of magnesia, etc., individually.

Laboratory charges are enumerated study by study, not by the tube of blood. Each blood drawing may call for five to fifty studies. You'll rarely know what they were or how many there were until you see your bill with its six pages of laboratory charges.

There is no possible way for any of us to keep track of and check these daily charges. One would have to be a 100 percent healthy accountant, working every minute during his hospital stay and studying every single event and collecting costs and charges from the relevant department as he went along. There would be no time to rest or get well.

The few items that you can check are the major infrequent events—for example, room charges. You know whether you were in the hospital for five or ten days. If your bill reflects an incorrect length of stay, speak out. Similarly, you know whether or not you've had an operation; whether you were in intensive care; whether part of your stay was in the coronary care unit. Numbers of days, locations, operations are simple matters that everyone can and should check.

PAYING THE BILL

Now that you have reviewed your bill you are faced with the $64,000 question: Who will pay and how much? Most people faithfully assume that insurance is insurance. Whether their employer provides health insurance or they have their own, they naïvely take for granted that it will cover all, or almost all, of the hospital charges. Having never reviewed their policies, many people find out too late that they are wrong. Now they're personally stuck for a $5,000, or possibly a $50,000, bill.

"STANDARD" HEALTH INSURANCE POLICIES

There is no such thing as a "standard" policy. Whether you are covered by Blue Cross, Aetna, Hartford, Equitable, or one of the hundreds of others that write health insurance, the policies are as variable as sickness itself. They run the gamut from total 100 percent coverage to $20 per day (out of an average charge of $300 to $400). They may cover up to a million dollars, or they may terminate when you have exhausted $2,500—after only a week or two in the hospital. In other words, it behooves you as the insured, and as the one who will have to pay if your policy is inadequate, to read the policy carefully, check with your salesman or office personnel department, and be *certain* before you need it what kind of coverage you actually have.

Most of the large companies and the federal government provide rather complete health insurance benefits for their employees. Union bargaining usually demands a comprehensive health package. Many smaller companies may provide the bare minimum. Even if your coverage is with Blue Cross, the contracts they write are quite variable. Many company contracts are co-pay: the insurer may pay only 50 to 80 percent of the daily charges; you are responsible for the rest. Some have a hefty deductible: the insured may have to pay the first $500 to $2,000 before his insurance pays anything. We can't cover all of the variations—they are individually tailored and span all possibilities—so check your policy coverage.

MAJOR MEDICAL

A most important feature, which is frequently overlooked, is so-called "major medical." This is health insurance that protects against a single catastrophic loss from an accident or injury. Many standard health insurance policies have an upper limit after which insurance is terminated. It may be $2,500 or a million dollars, depending on the particular policy. If it is less than $100,000, you should consider having a supplemental major medical policy to pick up charges that go beyond that. These policies are relatively inexpensive since the chances of your using them are rather small. If your basic policy reaches $500,000 or a million dollars, it really has a major medical built right in. Many of the large companies do provide policies like these. A chronic illness, a serious automobile accident, or any major injury can rapidly exhaust even a large insurance policy. Major medical plans offer the comfort of knowing that even if catastrophe strikes, your family's finances won't be wiped out by medical costs.

MEDICARE

Medicare affords only partial protection against sickness-related financial losses. The total coverage is limited; therefore, most medium- and upper-income individuals elect to have a second coinsurance policy such as Blue Cross to pick up where Medicare leaves off, plus a major medical policy to protect against the economic ravages of a prolonged illness.

Medicare automatically takes effect for all of our senior citizens aged 65 and above. Coverage in some form lasts for 90 continuous hospital days. After that the patient must be out of the acute care facility or skilled nursing facility for 60 days, after which another 90-day insured interval may begin. In other words, coverage for 90 days, 60 days at home or in a low-skilled-care nursing home, then 90 more days of coverage and the cycle repeats.

The 90 days of coverage includes the following: the first 60 days are almost completely covered (except for a $144 deductible charge which the patient must pay); the next 30 days are covered partially—Medicare pays all but $36 per day, the patient (or another insurance policy like Blue Cross) pays the other $36.

In addition to his 90-day coverage, each Medicare recipient has a small nest-egg reserve fund. He or she is entitled to a life time total of 60 additional co-pay ($36 by the patient, the rest by Medicare) days. What this means is that a single hospitalization of 150 days would be covered as follows: the first 60 days completely (less the $144 deductible), the next 90 days at $36 per day for the patient. That would terminate this 60-day reserve forevermore. Thereafter the maximum covered period would be 90 days. One can also use these 60 "bonus" days in increments—10 now, 20 the next time, 5 the following time until the 60 have been exhausted. To pick up the $144 deductible the $36 per day co-pay and the expenses of a protracted hospital stay beyond 90 days, it is wise to carry additional insurance. Most of the major health insurance carriers have policies that are tailored to these needs of Medicare recipients.

If skilled nursing-home care in an acute care facility is required following hospitalization, Medicare will cover part of the bill assuming certain criteria are met. First, the patient must have a certificate of need, which is generally arranged by the hospital social worker. This certificate is granted by the local PSRO (Professional Standards Review Organization) or a health agency arm of the federal government. They review the patient's clinical situation and either accept or deny the application for Medicare coverage. In other words, they determine whether skilled nursing-home care is or is not needed. If coverage is granted, it is paid as follows: the first 20 days are fully covered; the next 80 days are co-pay—the patient pays $18 per day, the government pays the rest.

At the end of 100 days, coverage ends for that period. Just as in the hospital situation, the patient can leave the skilled nursing home and go home or to a relative's house for 60 days. If, after that time skilled nursing care is again mandatory—and accepted by the government agency—100 days of skilled nursing-home care can restart. This cycle of 100 continuous nursing-home days interrupted by 60 days in a low-skilled-care facility or at home can repeat indefinitely. Notice we have talked here about "skilled" nursing-home care. The designation is very important, for unless the nursing home is officially designated a "skilled" facility, Medicare won't pay. A skilled facility becomes so designated on the basis of the kinds of treatment it is prepared to provide, the number of RNs per number of patients, the types of nursing observations that are carried out, and the availability of physician staff on the premises or on call. (There is more detailed information on this in the next chapter.) The Medicare agency makes that determination.

Not all nursing homes are "skilled"; the admissions office, administrator, or local Medicare office can tell you. These are facilities that offer *some* level of sophisticated patient observation. It is important to clarify whether or not the nursing home is skilled or not. The reason: Medicare does not pay a cent for unskilled nursing homes, custodial facilities, standard old-age homes. In addition, before Medicare will pick up a nursing-home bill, it reviews a patient's problem to be sure that it agrees that "skilled" care is really necessary.

The elderly patient who moves back and forth from an acute care nursing facility to a hospital for a protracted time period is in a real financial bind unless she or he has additional (Blue Cross, etc.) coverage. A respite in a skilled-care nursing home doesn't count for the 60-out-of-hospital days needed to restart the 90-day hospital coverage. Similarly, 60 days in a regular hospital doesn't permit the Medicare recipient to restart the 100 days of allotted skilled nursing care. Therefore, if a patient spends 90 days in the hospital, has already used up the special 60-day extra lifetime reserve, goes to a skilled nursing home for 100 days, then back to the hospital, no part of the last hospital bill will be covered by Medicare. If that same patient stays in the hospital for 60 days and then returns to the skilled nursing home—out of luck again. The bill for the skilled nursing home won't be touched by Medicare. In each case the 60 days' hiatus must be spent at home or in a low-skilled nursing facility before Medicare hospital or skilled nursing home payments can resume.

❦

MEDICAID

Medicaid is the health care coverage underwritten by the federal government in conjunction with state agencies to care for the medically indigent. To qualify, the recipient must have an income at or well below the poverty level.

Medicaid payment systems are unbelievably complex. They vary from state to state and follow at least 50 different formulas. In one state it may pay full charges. In another it will pay $36 daily toward a hospital bill.

Because of the red tape involved with Medicaid forms, the length of time it takes for payment, and the usually nominal coverage provided, a few hospitals and some physicians (right or wrong) are unable or unwilling to accept Medicaid patients.

18

The Social Worker as a Member of the Health Care Team and a Guide to Posthospital Care

One of the least understood and, at certain times, most necessary and valuable services your hospital may provide is the guidance of the social services department to help you find solutions to a great variety of problems. Just as medical, surgical, and nursing care will vary from hospital to hospital, with the larger, best-equipped institutions having the biggest staffs, so too will the particular type of social services available vary (the social service department is a required service of all accredited hospitals).

AIDING THE PATIENT PSYCHOLOGICALLY, FINANCIALLY, ENVIRONMENTALLY, AND SOCIALLY

Since social workers view the patient as part of a family system, their services are available to both patients and their families. A patient may be seen alone, or with the other family members if it is desired. You, or a relative, may ask directly for such services; or the suggestion may come from a doctor, nurse, or other professional staff member.

The emotional burdens an illness places on everyone involved is often one of those areas where help is most needed. The patient's separation from his loved ones, from his job, from his community, may be difficult to bear. If the patient has always been the decision-maker in the family, his or her temporary absence may create additional problems when some other family member has to shoulder this responsibility. If the illness involved is a complex one, communication between the doctor, the patient, and the family may need some clarification and the help of an understanding and compassionate professional. In each of these cases a social worker may provide the kind of skilled intervention that can help alleviate emotional stress.

Financial worries are another problem the patient may encounter when he least needs it. The social worker can help refer the patient to the billing department of the hospital for a discussion of his financial situation if difficulties arise. Beyond that, social workers can counsel those who qualify for disability over a prolonged period of time. And they can guide the patient to the proper social security office to explore possible benefits. In addition, since programs vary from state to state, the social worker is the one to consult about any possible coverage for catastrophic illness. (For example, some states have "inpatient Medicaid" available to those who are not indigent but find themselves in a situation where their medical bills are exceeding one quarter of their annual net income, even after the insurance has been paid. The amount of coverage for this may depend on whatever financial resources are left.)

Posthospital care needs may involve both personnel and equipment. The social worker is your best source of information and can help you mobilize many community resources and explore possible Medicare or Blue Cross, Blue Shield coverage in each situation, if you qualify. We will list a few of these resources:

Visiting Nurses

Based on the recommendation of your physician you may require the services of a visiting nurse, an RN. She will then determine the frequency of her visits and the length of her stay (usually not more than half an hour). She may provide services such as teaching a diabetic to take insulin, helping him supervise his diet, changing his surgical dressings or Foley catheters, taking care of ostomies, or teaching relatives how to care for a patient's bedsores, to cite a few examples.

Home Health Aide

This is a part-time housekeeper who will offer such services as shopping, preparing light meals, straightening up, and helping to give baths. You may also be eligible for Medicare benefits for a home health aide, but only if you have a condition that also necessitates a visiting nurse.

Physical or Speech Therapist

If you have been receiving such therapy in the hospital, your doctor may want you to continue it. A hospital social worker is an excellent guide to such therapists within your own community, even if it is not in the same state.

Meals on Wheels

This organization provides one meal a day for house-bound individuals over sixty who have no homemaker. As the specifics may vary slightly from state to state, we suggest you check your local chapter.

Equipment

You may need to rent, on a temporary basis, such equipment as a hospital bed, wheelchair, or portable oxygen. The social worker can help you arrange either a rental or a purchase, based upon your coverage.

Whether your needs are for full-time twenty-four-hour care, a practical nurse, a home health aide, or suitable equipment, the social worker can refer you to the best agencies to handle your requirements.

Another area in which patients leaving the hospital after a major illness may require help involves improving the quality of their lives. A social worker can help such a patient find ways to socialize through such community programs as recreation centers and senior citizen centers. Even after your discharge, you and/or your family may want to see a social worker on a more regular basis to work on any difficulties in adjusting to your illness.

HELPING PATIENTS CHOOSE THE APPROPRIATE AFTER-CARE FACILITY

For those patients who aren't able to return home immediately after they leave the hospital, either because they require an additional period of convalescence or because they live alone, an after-care facility may be the answer. The social worker will meet with patient, doctor, nurses, or therapists involved, assess the patient's needs, and then, together with the patient and the family, initiate a plan of action. Here is a list of a few of the after-care facilities which may be available:

Rehabilitation Centers

These are hospitals with a highly trained staff of rehabilitation workers, consisting of specialized physicians; nurses; social workers; speech, physical, and occupational therapists, capable of working with patients who have various degrees of handicaps. These centers are designed to reeducate and retrain such patients to achieve the maximum level of independent functioning. He may stay for a few weeks or a few months depending on treatment goals. Most of these facilities have inpatient and outpatient services so that the patient can continue therapy even after he or she has improved enough to return to the community. If you have a disability that prevents you from returning to your former line of work, you may want to see a rehabilitation counselor to explore retraining for a job you are better able to handle.

Chronic Disease Hospitals

These manage patients with nonrehabilitative disorders, such as terminal illnesses, severe chronic obstructive lung disease (emphysema, black lung disease of coal miners), medication-dependent asthma, progressive or static neurologic diseases (coma, brain injuries), disabilities requiring tube feedings, or constant intravenous solutions.

Skilled Nursing Facilities

These are nursing homes. They admit patients who need twenty-four-hour nursing care. In many communities, patients requiring care at chronic disease hospitals would be cared for here. These patients are generally recovering from problems such as strokes, severe diabetes, recent orthopedic surgery (hip fractures, long-term casting), readjustment of medication for Parkinson's disease. Your length of stay may vary from a short to an extended period.

Intermediate Level Nursing Homes

These health-related facilities help patients who cannot manage for themselves and continue to need nursing and medical supervision. To qualify it is necessary to be ambulatory. The patients in these homes usually suffer from senile disorders, severe arthritis, disorders involving hardening of the arteries.

Domiciliary Facilities

These are for fully independent patients who can manage for themselves but need supervision of medications, special diets, help with meals, and someone available should their condition deteriorate. One or more nurses are generally on the premises and a doctor is on call.

Hospices

These are for patients with terminal cancer or other fatal disorders. This type of facility is relatively new in the United States but a longtime fixture in England. It is designed to help the patient and the family through this painful, emotionally disruptive time. The personnel are trained in the management of death and dying, with special emphasis on resolution of emotional conflicts and relief of pain.

Terminal Care Facilities

These can be synonymous with hospices; other times they designate care of terminal cases other than cancer. As both facilities are fairly new, we suggest you check with your social services department.

Private insurance may cover a portion of the expenses incurred in some of these facilities. This will depend upon the type of insurance contract and the level of care required. Medicare insurance will cover a limited number of days, but only in a skilled-nursing facility and provided you enter within fourteen days after hospital discharge.

In these pages we have attempted to offer you a useful guide to the often confusing and sometimes frightening world of hospitals. Our intended audience includes all prospective and current patients: you, your friends, your relatives. We can't afford to ignore the hospital world for, like it or not, nearly all of us will someday be patients. We strongly believe that thorough information gathering and thoughtful preparation will help ensure your comfort, safety, and peace of mind when that day arrives.

We have tried to provide practical advice, general guidelines, and currently available resources to help you make a rational and proper choice of a hospital. We've give you useful information to help you get along once you're there. We sincerely hope and believe that fortifying you with this knowledge will make your hospital stay a positive experience, one that is likely to reward you with a favorable, healthful outcome.

Index

A

Accommodations, basic points
    about, 72–73
Accredited hospitals, 42
Aches, postsurgical, 159
Admission to hospital,
    expediting, 70–77
  elective admissions, 71–76
    accommodations, basic
      points about, 72–73
    admitting office,
      information needed and
      how to supply it, 73–74
    bringing work with you, 75
    routine testing, 71–72
    timesaving tips, 75–76
    what to bring with you,
      74–75
    when not insured, 76
  emergency, 76–77
    children, 189–90
  patient checklist, 77
Admitting office, information
    needed and how to
    supply it, 73–74

After-care facilities, 203–6
Ambulance services, 45, 47–48
American Hospital Association,
    60
Amputations, 33–34
Anesthesia
    caliber of the practice of, 22
    general, 19, 21
    local, 19
    as most dangerous aspect of
      surgery, 21–24
    the surgeon and, 20
Anesthesiologists, 22–24
    preoperative visit by, 149–50
Anesthesiology, 22
Anesthetists, 21–24
    nurse, 23
Angiographic studies, 126
Antacid medications, 157
Appetite, postsurgical, 155–56
Arteriography, 27
Arts and crafts services, 178
Assessing your needs, 15–35,
    88–92
    finding out about hospitals,
      27–28

levels of care, 34–35
    routine care, 19–20
      hospital, 19–20
      outpatient, 19
    second-level medical
      problems, 26
    second-level surgical care,
      21–26
      judging competence of
        surgeon, 24–25
      nursing care following
        surgery, 25
      protection from most
        dangerous aspect of
        surgery, 21–24
    special care needs, 31–34
    third-level medical care, 29–
      30
    third-level surgical care and
      procedures, 28–29
Autologous blood transfusions,
    128
B
Backache, postsurgical, 159
Bacteriologic examinations, 125
Barbiturates, 138

Baylor University, 40
Blood tests, 123
Blood transfusions, 128
Blue Cross, 71, 195–98
  unwarranted hospitalization
    and, 19
Blue Shield, 62
Board-certified surgeons, 25
Board-eligible surgeons, 25
Bone-marrow studies, 124
Bookmobiles, 178
Bradley method, 135, 136
Bronchography, 27
Burn centers, 166

C

California, University of, 38, 39
Caring For Your Unborn Child
    (Gots and Gots), 135
CAT scanner, 126–27
Cesarean sections, 144–45
Children
  emergency admissions, 189–
    90
  emergency departments, 59–
    60
  helping child recover, 190–91
  preparing for the hospital,
    180–91
    changing child's doctor,
      184–85
    in the hospital, 187–89
    selecting the hospital, 183–
      84
    your own preparation,
      181–83
  special care needs, 31–33
Children's hospitals, 41
Choosing a hospital,
    importance of, 4–14
  differences in hospitals, 10–
    12
  making the decision, 12–14
Chronic disease hospitals, 204
Cleveland Clinic, 40, 41
Columbia University, 38, 39
Comfort in the hospital, 86–88
Common sense, 17, 146
Complaints
  against nurses
    major, 90–92
    minor, 89–90
  against physician staff, 99
  emergency department,
    55–57

Complete blood count (CBC),
    123
Constipation, postsurgical,
    157–59
Coronary artery bypass
    operation, 40–41
Coronary care units (CCUs),
    167–68
Cytology, 125–26

D

Demerol, 138
Domiciliary facilities, 204–5
Drugs, labor and delivery, 138–
    39
Duke University, 38, 39

E

Elderly patients, the nurse and,
    92
Elective admissions, 71–76. *See
    also* Admission to
    hospital
Emergencies, 44–62
  admission, 76–77
  children, 189–90
  ambulance services, 45, 47–
    48
  assessing attention problem
    deserves, 51–54
  first-aid courses, 45
  health insurance, 62
  hospital away from home,
    65–68
    arranging a transfer, 66–68
  how to decide whom to call,
    46–48
  planning ahead for, 44–46
  poison-control lists, 44–45
  telephone numbers, 45, 47
Emergency departments, 44–62
  children, 59–60
  dissatisfaction with
    treatment, 60–62
  how to expedite care, 54–55
  making your complaints
    heard, 55–57
  misusing, 62
  priorities of, 51–53
  psychology of personnel of,
    49–51
  researching, 45–46
  roles visitors can play in
    emergency care, 57–59
  understanding, 48
  what to demand from, 54–55

Environmental aid, 200–203
Episiotomy, 142
Evaluating hospitals, 36–43
  general data, 36–37
  miscellaneous methods of,
    42–43
  nonteaching hospitals, 42
  teaching hospitals, 37–39
    finding the best, 39–41
  university hospitals, 37–39

F

Family's role, special care units,
    169–70
Female physicians, 15
Financial aid, 200–203
First-aid courses, 45
Food, hospital, 175–77

G

Galton, Lawrence, 157–58
Gas pains, postsurgical, 157–59
Gifts, 179
Gots, B. A., 135
Gots, R. E., 135

H

Handicapped patients, the
    nurse and, 92–93
Harvard University, 38, 39
Health insurance, 71–72
  Blue Cross, 71, 195–98
    unwarranted
      hospitalization and, 19
  Blue Shield, 62
  emergencies, 62
  lack of, 76
  major medical, 196
  Medicaid, 73, 199
  Medicare, 73, 196–99
  standard, 195–96
  unwarranted hospitalization
    and, 19
Hiccups, postsurgical, 159
Hip replacement, 33–34
Histology, 125–26
Home health aide, 202
Hospices, 205
Hospital food, 175–77
Hospitals away from home, 63–
    69
  emergencies, 65–68
    arranging a transfer, 66–68
  illness in the hotel, 69
  illness while abroad, 69

preplanning, 68–69
Hotels, illness in, 69
Hypnosis, 135

I

Insomnia, postsurgical, 156
Intensive care units (ICUs),
    166–67
Intermittent positive pressure
    breathing apparatus
    (IPPB) 129, 161
International Childbirth
    Education Association
    (CEA), 135–37
Intestinal cramps, postsurgical,
    157–59

J

John Hopkins University
    Hospital, 38, 50, 167
Joint Commission on
    Accreditation of
    Hospitals (JCAH), 3,
    42–43, 96

L

Labor and delivery, 131–42
    Cesarean sections, 144–45
    drugs, 138–39
    finding physician sharing
        goals, 136–37
    home versus hospital, 131–34
    natural childbirth, 135, 136
    new alternatives, 134–36
    procedures, 141–42
        episiotomy, 142
    selecting obstetrician and
        obstetrical hospital,
        139–41
Laboratory studies and
        procedures, 122–30
    bacteriologic examinations,
        125
    blood tests, 123
    cytology, 125–26
    histology, 125–26
    miscellaneous, 124
    nuclear medicine, 126–27
    radiology, 126–27
    spinal taps, 124–25
    techniques and equipment,
        128–30
        blood transfusions, 128
        respiratory assistive
            devices, 128–29

tubes, 129–30
    urinalysis, 123, 124
Lamaze method, 135, 136
Laughing gas, 138
Leaving the hospital, 192–99
    major medical health
        insurance, 196
    Medicaid, 199
    Medicare, 196–99
    paying the bill, 195
    reviewing the bill, 193–94
    standard health insurance,
        195–96
Leboyer, Dr., 134–36
Levels of care, 34–35
Licensed practical nurses
    (LPNs), 79, 81
Local nursing associations, 43
Local rescue squads, 43

M

M. D. Anderson Hospital, 41
Massachusetts General
    Hospital, 16
Mayo Clinic, 39
Meals on wheels, 202
Medicaid, 73, 199
Medical intensive care unit
    (MICU), 167
Medical students, advantages
    of being examined by,
    105–7
Medicare, 73, 196–99
Michigan, University of, 38, 39
Mistakes, minimizing, 118–20
Morphine, 138
Myelography, 27

N

Natural childbirth, 135, 136
Nausea, postsurgical, 155
Neighborhood (community)
    hospitals, 15–16
Neonatal intensive care units
    (NICUs), 169
Neurological injury units, 166
Nitrous oxide, 138
Nonsurgical conditions, 20
Nonteaching hospitals
    evaluating, 42
        physician staff, 99–103
        role of consultants, 102–3
Nuclear medicine, 126–27
Nurse-midwives, 83

Nurses
    achieving a more effective
        relationship, 84–95
    assessing needs, 88–92
    comfort, 86–88
    elderly patients, 92
    handicapped patients, 92–
        93
    major complaints, 90–92
    minor complaints, 89–90
    private-duty nurses, 93–95
    safety, 86–88
    anesthetists, 23
    care following surgery, 25
    hierarchy of, 79–81
    licensed practical (LPNs), 79,
        81
    nurse-midwives, 83
    nursing aides (NAs), 81
    ostomy, 83
    practical, 43
    private-duty, 82–83
        achieving a more effective
            relationship, 93–95
        postsurgical patient and,
            160
    registered (RNs), 43, 79–81
    understanding, 78–83
    university hospitals, 38
    visiting, 201–2
Nursing aides (NA), 81
Nursing associations, local, 43
Nursing homes, 204

O

Obstetrical hospitals, selecting,
    139–41
Obstetricians, selecting, 139–41
Operations. See Surgery
Orthopedic surgeons, 34
Ostomy nurses, 83
Outpatient care, routine, 19

P

Pain, postsurgical, 154–55, 159
Pap smear, 123
Patient checklist, 77
Patient education, special, 83,
    177–78
Patient orientation, 174–75
Pennsylvania, Univeristy of, 38,
    39
Physical therapists, 202

Physician care in hospital, 109–21
 special requests, 118–21
  to examining physician, 118
  minimizing mistakes, 118–20
  when and how to change doctors, 120–21
 team approach, whom to talk to, 116–17
 well-coordinated, 115–16
Physician staff, 96–108
 chain of command, 97–99
 complaints against, 99
 nonteaching hospitals, 99–103
 role of consultants, 102–3
 the professional hierarchy, 98
 teaching hospitals, 103–8
  advantages of examination by medical student, 105–7
  coordination of care, 107–8
  understanding role of physicians, 104–5
Physicians
 changing your child's, 184–85
 choosing, 17
 credentials of, 17
 female, 15
 understanding role of, 104–5
 university-based, 38
 who shares goals in childbirth, 136–37
Pneumoencephalography, 27
Poison-control lists, 44–45
Posthospital care. See Social workers (posthospital care)
Postsurgical discomfort. See Surgery, postsurgical discomfort
Practical nurses, 43
Pre-admission testing (P.A.T.), 71
Private nurses, 82–83
 achieving a more effective relationship, 93–95
 postsurgical patient and, 160
Private room versus roommates, 173–74
Professional Standards Review Organization (PSRO), 3, 197

Psychological aid, 200–203

Q
Quality Care Management Consultants, 3
Questions about daily hospital life, 171–79
 arts and crafts services, 178
 bookmobiles, 178
 gifts, 179
 hospital food, 175–77
 patient orientation, 174–75
 relatives sleeping in, 178
 roommates versus private room, 173–74
 special patient education, 177–78
 visiting hours, 171–73
 visitors, 171–73
Quinlan, Karen Ann, 129

R
Radioactive scanning, 127
Radioisotope scanning, 127
Radiology, 126–27
Registered nurses (RNs), 43, 79–81
Rehabilitation centers, 203–4
Relatives sleeping in, 178
Renal dialysis centers, 168
Rescue squads, local, 43
Respiratory assistive devices, 128–29
Roommates versus private room, 173–74
Roswell Park Hospital, 41

S
Safety in the hospital, 86–88
Save Your Stomach (Galton), 157–58
Serology, 123
Shock-trauma centers, 165–66
Sloan Kettering Hospital, 41
Social aid, 200–203
Social workers (posthospital care), 200–206
 after-care facilities, 203–6
 chronic disease hospitals, 204
 domiciliary facilities, 204–5
 environmental aid, 200–203
 equipment, 202–3
 financial aid, 200–203
 home health aide, 202
 hospices, 205

meals on wheels, 202
 nursing homes, 204
 physical therapist, 202
 psychological aid, 200–203
 rehabilitation centers, 203–4
 social aid, 200–203
 speech therapist, 202
 terminal care facilities, 205
 visiting nurses, 201–2
Special care needs, 31–34
 amputations, 33–34
 children, 31–33
 hip replacement, 33–34
Special care units, 163–70
 burn centers, 166
 coronary care units (CCUs), 167–68
 family's role, 169–70
 intensive care units (ICUs), 166–67
 neonatal intensive care units (NICUs), 169
 neurological injury units, 166
 renal dialysis centers, 168
 shock-trauma centers, 165–66
Specialists, 30
Speech therapists, 202
Spinal tap, 124–25
Stanford University Medical Center, 41
Superspecialists, 30
Surgeons
 anesthesia and, 20
 board-certified, 25
 board eligible, 25
 judging competence of, 24–25
 orthopedic, 34
Surgery, 143–62
 assisting with your recovery, 160–61
 Cesarean sections, 144–45
 close postoperative attendance, 21
 common sense approach, 146
 day of surgery, 151–52
 first day in hospital, 147–48
 guide to various operations, 162
 immediately following, 152
 most dangerous aspect of, protection from, 21–24
 postsurgical discomfort, 152–55
  aches and pains, 154–55, 159

backache, 159
constipation, 157–59
gas pains, 157–59
hiccups, 159
insomnia, 156
intestinal cramps, 157–59
nausea, 155
pain, 154–55, 159
private-duty nurses, 160
regaining appetite, 155–56
urination, 156–57
vomiting, 155
prehospitalization
  discussions, 145–47
preoperative visit by the
  anesthesiologist, 149–50
standard, 16
the surgical "prep," 150–51
Surgical care
protection from most
  dangerous aspect of
  surgery, 21–24
second-level, 21–26
  judging competence of
    surgeon, 24–25
  nursing care following
    surgery, 25
third-level, 28–29
Surgical intensive care unit
  (SICU), 167

T

Teaching hospitals, 37–39
  evaluating, 37–39

finding the best, 39–41
physician staff, 103–8
  advantages of examination
    by medical student,
    105–7
  coordination of care, 107–8
  understanding role of
    physicians, 104–5
Team approach, whom to talk
  to, 116–17
Telephone numbers,
  emergency, 45, 47
Terminal care facilities, 205
Testing
  pre-admission (P.A.T.), 71
  routine, 71–72
  X-ray, 71, 126
Tests
  blood, 123
  level-three procedures, 27
  level-two procedures, 27–28
  routine, 20
  special, 27
  specialized, 29
Texas Heart Institute, 40, 41
Therapists
  physical, 202
  speech, 202
Tibbits, Samuel J., 60
Tranquilizers, 138
Travel, hospitals away from
  home, 63–69
  emergencies, 65–68
    arranging a transfer, 66–68

illness in the hotel, 69
illness while abroad, 69
preplanning, 68–69
Tubes, 129–30

U

University hospitals,
  evaluating, 37–39
University of Maryland
  Hospital, 165
Urinalysis, 123, 124
Urination, postsurgical, 156–57

V

Valium, 138
Vanderbilt University, 38, 39
Visiting hours, 171–73
Visting nurses, 201–2
Visitors, 171–73
  in emergency care, 57–59
Vomiting, postsurgical, 155

W

Washington Hospital Center,
  39
Washington University, 39
Work, bringing to hospital with
  you, 75

X

X-ray testing, 71, 126

Y

Yale University, 38, 39